I0455561

This Book is dedicated to my children, my husband and to the amazing women who inspired me to write this book.

Embracing Birth:

A Collection of Inspiring Birth Stories

Jessica L. Levesque

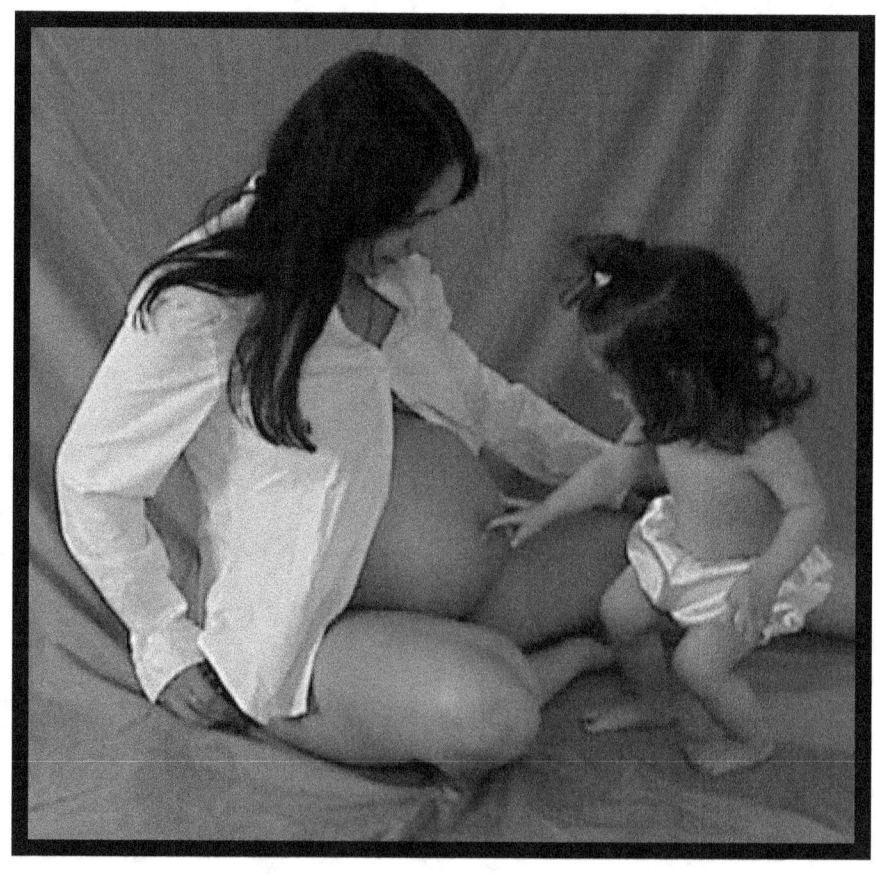

No part of this book may be reproduced in any form,

by any means, without written permission from the author.

Copyright 2008

Embracing Birth: A Collection of Inspiring Birth Stories

Jessica L. Levesque

Thank you for purchasing this book.

Introduction

I am honored to have collected many amazing and inspiring birth stories. They are all put together in this fantastic book with many beautiful pictures. I believe with all of my heart that women's bodies were made perfectly to give birth. Women have a great opportunity to be empowered through experiencing childbirth in a loving supportive environment, surrounded by people who believe in them and their ability to birth. I have seen first hand the amazing abilities of the female body. My wish is that everyone is able to make educated decisions regarding their rights and choices for childbirth. I wish you many blessings on your journey to parenthood.

Acknowledgements

Thank you to all of the mothers that contributed birth stories to Embracing Birth. Your trust and faith in yourself and in your body made this book possible. I am very grateful to you. May you continue to live your life with strength and inner guidance. Thank you to my family for allowing me the time to read hundreds of birth stories, along with compiling and editing this book. To my husband Greg, thank you for providing me the space needed to complete this book. I am very grateful. Thanks mom. Thank you, Jewel and Kaden for being my inspiration for this book. Thank you to all midwives, doulas, other birth professionals, advocates and mothers who believe that birth is a normal natural process.

We have a secret in our culture...
and it's not that birth is painful. It's that women are strong."
- Laura Stavoe Harm

Embracing Birth: A Collection of Inspiring Birth Stories

Table of Contents

Page

Dedication ………………………………………………………….…… 1

Introduction…………………………………………………………...…..4

Acknowledgements…………………………………………………….…4

Hospital Births..9

Jeweliana Rose…………………………………………………………...…10

Sapphire Lynn…………………………………………………………….16

Sean Edward and Seth Thomas……………………………...……………...19

Ayla…………………………………………………………………………25

Charles Henry…………………………………………………….…………27

Birth Center Births………………………………………..………………**32**

Alex and Andre……………………………………………………………...33

Nicholas Raymond…………………………………………………………35

Home births…………………………………………………..36

Alejandro David………………………………………….37

Carson Moss…………………………………………...45

Gabriel Ryan…………………………………………..49

Kaian Gregory……………………………………...62

Matthew……………………………………………..68

Ryan……………………………………………….71

Ellyse Quinn…………………………………………...82

Jordyn Rose…………………………………………....88

Soterius…………………………………………...96

Linkin Alexander…………………………………….97

Maeve…………………………………………….....101

Sophia…………………………………………........107

Eva Robin…………………………………………....124

Morgan Marie………………………………………...131

Twins…………………………………………….134

Solomon …………………………………………...143

Laurel Anne…………………………………………147

Aurora…………………………………………….154

ChristoFinn………………………………………...156

Violet Hope………………………………………………………..…166

Morvryn Sage………………………………………………….……..177

Gianna Belle…………………………………………………….……186

Anayi and Eliyah………………………………………..…..…….…...192

Kaden Reece………………………………………………...….……..205

About the Author……………………………………………….……213

Creating your birth…………………………………………….……...214

Afterward……………………………………………………….……216

Resources……………………………………………………….……219

Hospital Births

Jeweliana Rose

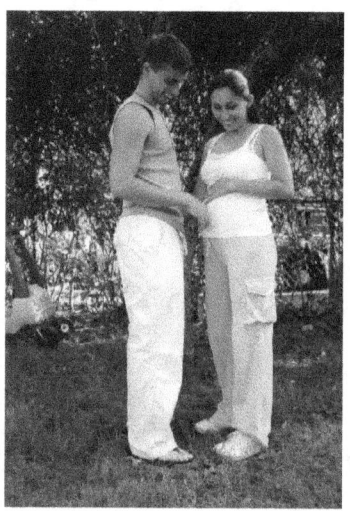

It was cold winter night in New England. I had insomnia and was working very hard with my husband Gregory to finish the baby's nursery. I had contractions that had started at 36 weeks. We had been in a car accident with a deer when we were traveling to Florida and since our car was totaled we had to take an airplane home. The flight restarted the contractions and they continued every five minutes until my water broke at 39 ½ weeks. We finished the nursery at 3:30 a.m. and I fell asleep on the couch. Two hours later at 5:30 a.m. my water broke. It was just a trickle but it woke me and I got up and went straight to the bathroom to check. I knew it was time so I went upstairs and woke up my husband Greg. I was so excited my baby was on her way. I called the midwives office and they said they would page the midwife. We hung around for a little bit.

I was so tired but so happy that soon the contractions would be over and I'd be holding a baby girl in my arms.

We already had the car packed and ready to go so off we went. Of course my dear husband had to stop for coffee first. We drove to Women and Infants hospital in Rhode Island. We arrived around 6:30 a.m. I was admitted to triage and checked, I was 2 cm dilated.

My sister Stephanie arrived before I was sent to the Alternative Birthing Center. We went down a few floors to the ABC. The nurse welcomed us and suggested a shower. I had met her a few times before and was happy to see a familiar face. My sister and the nurse tried to find the right temperature for the water. I held on to the bar in the shower and stomped my feet and was doing deep breathing. The contractions were very close they felt wonderful and I was so excited. I felt very confident in my ability to handle this challenge and was filled with energy. I was feeling so happy.

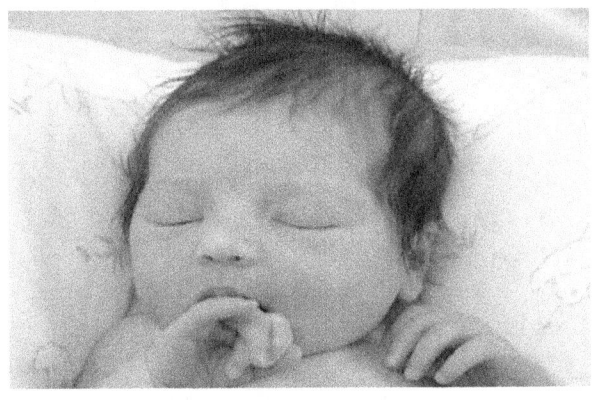

Then my nurse asked if I would like to try the bath, so they started filling the large whirlpool tub for me. The birth room was very large and was setup like a bedroom. It had a private bathroom with a shower. There was a large living room/waiting area right through the birthing room. It also has a shared bathroom with a large whirlpool tub which was dark green. Everyone had now arrived. My best friend Sharon who was my doula, my dad, and my mother, father, sister and brother in-laws were all there. The midwife who I hadn't met yet had not arrived because they had paged an off duty midwife and it took them awhile to figure this out.

I emerged myself nude into the hot water and felt so much relief followed by intense unrelenting contractions. I thought the contractions were supposed to start and stop but they didn't; it was wave after wave. There were many women huddled into the bathroom now. A midwife in training had arrived but no midwife, whom I really wouldn't have noticed; I was quite involved in the waves. I was far away in labor land and it had only been a few hours.

I got out of the tub and walked around some more, than I tried to lean on and push down on Greg, but he was too tall. So I put my arms around my sister Stephanie who is my height and pushed her down as hard as I could. It felt so good to push down. I felt like I needed to go to the bathroom so I did. I than remembered I wanted to try different positions. So I went down on all fours and that lasted one second. All I could feel was the baby so very low and anything but being upright felt unnatural. I went back into the tub and then it became unbearable. I wanted it to be over with I didn't want to do it anymore. I thought this was just the beginning, how would I last 10 more hours of this intensity. I said, "I can't do this." and my friend Sharon said, "You are doing this." as she put a washcloth on my face.

The water wasn't helping me relax anymore and I felt I needed to walk around again. Sharon put in my meditation cd for me. Sharon is the kind of person you want around you when you are in this state of mind. She had complete trust and faith in me. I knew she would protect me if needed, so that I would always remember my experience with love. The midwife just arrived. I said, "I think I want to go upstairs and get an epidural if this is going to go on" My husband had told the nurses without me knowing to ignore my request for pain medication. He knew how important it was to me to have a natural childbirth. The nurse said, "Well let's check you and see how far you are" So I reached down and I felt Jeweliana's head crowning. I said, "I can feel her head!" I was so excited my mood changed instantly. I was almost done! Oh the joy in my heart.

The nurse asked me to lay down on the queen size bed. Then they set me up with pillows behind me. I did want to squat for pushing but at that moment I had forgotten and I was too excited. I had a huge smile on my face. I had my sister Stephanie on one side of me, my husband Greg on the other side with all the other women in the room surrounding the bed. Greg was going to catch the baby. With one contraction as I was waiting for them to get situated with the birthing supplies I pushed him and the nightstand he sat on a few feet away with ease. Now I was ready to push and I meant business. I had a foolish idea in my head of woman

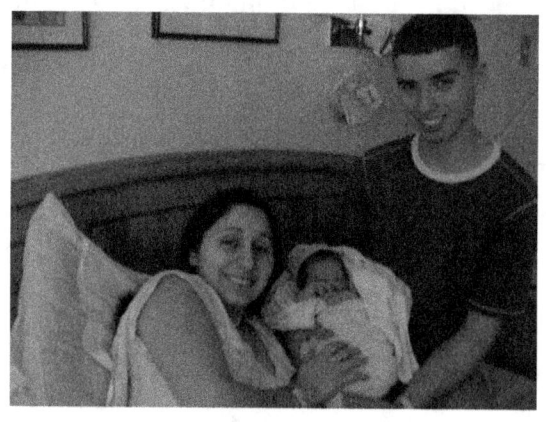

pushing for hours (silly me). I thought well that is not going to be me. This baby is coming out now. So Greg went to the bottom of the bed to catch the baby. The midwife and midwife in training were behind him in blue scrubs and funny shields on their faces. They applied a hot compress to my perineum. I pushed once and felt her head come out and slide back in. I said, "Oh no baby you're coming out" and I pushed through the ring of fire and her head came out. I felt the warm gush of fluids rush out over me, and that felt wonderful. Greg didn't expect that and now he knew why the midwives had those silly shields. With another breath I pushed her body out and Greg handed her to me. Jeweliana Rose was born at 9:54 a.m. 4 hours and 24 minutes after my water broke. "There she is my baby" I said softly. I nursed her immediately and left the cord intact until it was done pulsating. She had a head full of dark hair just like I had dreamed she did.

The midwife gave me pitocin to deliver the placenta. I didn't want that but I was so involved in Jeweliana I didn't take notice at the time. She then stitched up my tears. The whole baby in and out thing has a nice gradual purpose that I didn't allow to happen. I was overwhelmed with love and joy for my little angel. What an incredibly amazing experience it was. I was overjoyed. I held her and held her and than her daddy got another chance to hold her. Everyone left and we stayed in the ABC for about three hours after her birth. Greg and I just laid in the bed together holding our baby, marveling over her beauty.

I couldn't sleep at all I was filled with so much incredible energy. I was amazed at what had just happened and how it all went so fast. At 3:00 a.m. my husband and baby who stayed right in my arms were sleeping I woke up around 9:00 a.m. When we went home I was finally able to sleep comfortably and fully enjoy my baby. All I could do was hold her. Having a baby inside you for so long and than there she is; that is so amazing. She is such a blessing and I am very grateful to have such a healthy beautiful little girl.

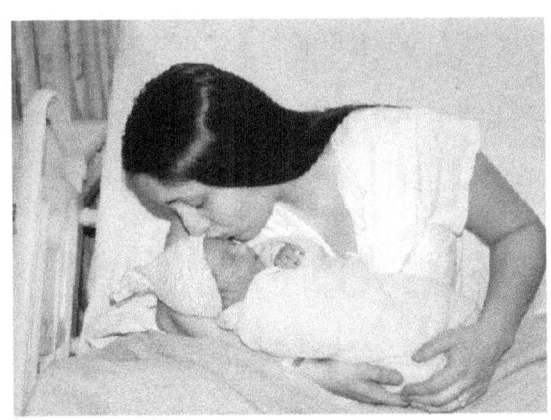 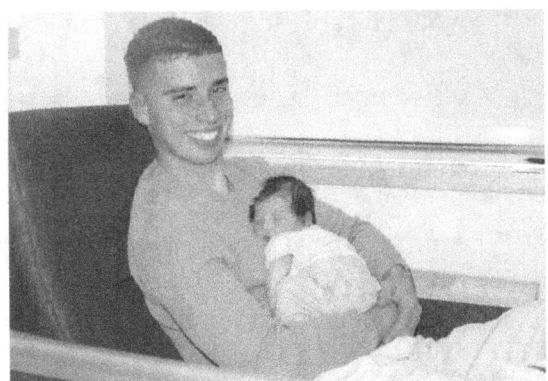

Mommy	: Jessica Levesque
Daddy	: Greg Levesque
City State	: Providence RI
Age at birth	: 21
Birth	: First
Baby's name	: Jeweliana Rose
Baby's height	: 19 1/4 inches
Baby's weight	: 6lbs 4oz

Sapphire

1989 I found out I was pregnant. I was presently surprised to hear this news. I did not give any thought to whether I wanted to have natural childbirth or not. My pregnancy went well I stayed relatively small throughout my pregnancy. I was very active and did not like to be babied.

On December 27th 1989 I awoke early to use the bathroom, I discovered that I had lost my plug and labor would soon follow. I was too excited to sleep so I awoke a friend that was staying with me and told them my news. I had lots of energy and cleaned and tidied the house for hours knowing this would be the last I would be able to do before the baby would be coming home. I called the Doctors office once I knew they would be open. They stated that because I had no contractions that I didn't need to be seen. I would need to wait until the contractions started and then come in when they were coming at regular intervals. I was home all day waiting for the big moment. It wasn't until 8:00 p.m. that I checked in with the hospital.

Once at the Hospital I was put in bed and told to relax and that they would be monitoring my progress. I stayed in bed for about 40 minutes and my contractions became further apart. I told them I wanted to get up and walk around, because until I got to the hospital I had been active and that I thought that moving about might help. So I walked up and down the stairs and throughout the hallway for about two hours until my water broke. At which point the pain increased and became more frequent. So at that point I was helped to my room to deal with my discomfort in the privacy of my own room.

I spent my time in the room on my hands and knees, and showering trying to relieve the back pain. After a few hours of this I was told to get in bed and try to sleep between the contractions. I thought that they were crazy but I actually was able to get some rest. As the baby progressed in the birthing canal it got to the point of it being unbearable to be in bed on my back or on my bum. The nurse suggested that I go into the bathroom and sit on the toilet to relieve the pressure, naturally allowing the baby's head to crown. I felt very weird about this trip to the bathroom so close to the birth of my unborn baby, but once I sat down I was aware right away why this position was encouraged at this stage of labor. Within minutes my baby's head was showing and I was at the perfect angle to push. I leaned back against the wall and scooted my bum to the edge of the bowl, as a friend supported me as I pushed. I believe I pushed about 4-5 times and my baby was born. What a beautiful baby!

When it was time to push the birth was so quick. The pain was over right away to be left with discomfort. The whole process is amazing, inspiring, powerful, moving and even better that there were no drugs involved to interfere with this most cherished time in my life!

Mom	:Sharon L. Peck
Dad	:Ray C. Peck
City/State	:Randolph, Vermont
Age at birth	:19
Birth	:First
Baby's Name	:Sapphire Lynn
Baby's Length	:21 inches long
Baby's Height	:5'10 lbs

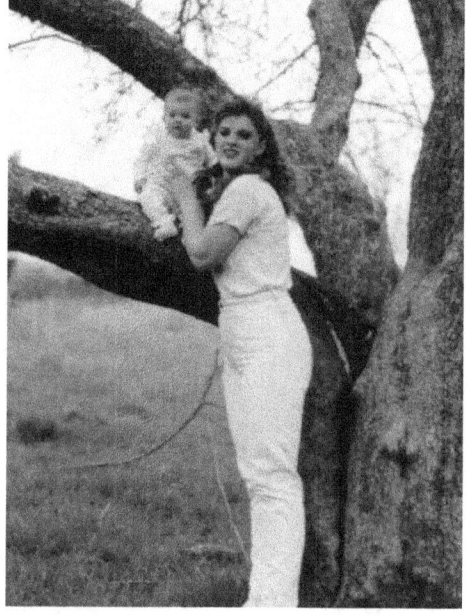

Sean Edward and Seth Thomas

This is how I created my first-time mother, drug-free vaginal twin birth. I guess it starts with my pre-natal's. I understand and even accept that twin births can simply go in the wrong direction in a very short amount of time. Once I found out at 20 weeks I was having twins, I chose to give up my homebirth plans and deal with the medical world.

I guess my attitude was; if it isn't broke, don't touch me. The nearest hospital to me only does c-sections for twins. So we went an extra forty minutes away to one that would be open to vaginal delivery. I was recommended a doctor who also has experience and was willing to deliver the second twin vaginally even if breech.

We got along all right, but every time I saw him, he brought up an epidural. Even after I told him the subject was no longer allowed to be discussed. I switched to another doctor at 32 weeks in the same clinic. He didn't have a type A personality and also was willing to catch my babies in a position other than flat on my back on the skinny metal non-negotiable OR table.

Let's fast forward to 35 weeks, 5 days pregnant. My homebirth midwife was now my doula and advocate. We had planned to drive the 1 1/2 hours and check into a Comfort Suites with a Jacuzzi than I would labor there next to the hospital. She would meet us at the hospital when things were really going. But instead, my waters broke at home at five in the morning. Instead, I just called her on the phone and we went for plan B. This was to labor at home for awhile, eat, and then get to the hospital hopefully later than sooner. I found the idea of being continually monitored and not allowed to eat offensive and wanted to delay it as long as possible.

I also was using the Hypnobabies program in hopes of having a pain-free birthing experience. It's hard for me to say what parts of it worked for me. I know I did not have a pain-free birthing. But time was in a warp speed all day and I was very calm and fearless the whole time. The first-stage was so easy. It was as bad as kind of annoying menstrual cramps. My husband and I used the Contraction Master (www.contractionmaster.com) and just packed and prepared. My water wouldn't stop leaking though and it eventually started to show some bloody show. That was good news that this was the real thing and would mean less interference from the docs.

The ride in the car wasn't that great. I tried to relax and listen to my Hypnobabies tapes, but I had to keep my muscles tight for all the moving the car was doing while on my hands and knees in the back seat. I gave up and just focused through the contractions. They were getting more intense, but quickly went away.

We got to the hospital at 1:30 p.m. and were astonished to find we were at 5 cm. I lied to them about when my water broke and said 11:00 a.m. knowing they put you 'on the clock'. My midwife/doula was called and showed up at 3:00 p.m. All the while, I just would look at the pretty black spruce out the window of the labor and delivery room during a contraction and breathe through it. Even though we had progressed beyond annoying menstrual cramps to more of a clamping down pain, it was easy to get through them and afterwards I'd just pick up my conversation where it left off.

Eventually I started to feel pushy. My body was doing it, not me! My midwife was surprised, but thought we should get checked and it turned out I was over 9 cm by 5:00 p.m. This is when the coolest thing happened. The labor and delivery nurse on hand informed me she would now wheel me down to OR in the birthing bed. My jaw dropped and I said, "Really? I fought with two different doctors over this subject!" She said, "Your doctor didn't forbid it, did he?" I thought quickly and carefully carved my sentence, "No. He forbade doing a C-section on a birth bed. He said it was too unsafe." He actually said he has no problem with birth beds, but the chance of c-section means they can't be used. She relaxed and said, "Oh that would never happen. We have an OR table on standby we would put you in." I remember thanking her right after the birth saying getting the birth bed was just like Christmas.

We get to the OR room and it's time to push. I definitely had the urge to push with the contractions, but there were only two urges at a time. It took me an awful long time to figure out how to make the most out of them. My husband and my doula were amazing, especially since the nurse wanted me to go into the infamous knees to your ears position for pushing. I looked at her like she was on crack and my doula, who has helped over 1800 babies birth in their own homes, knew she had to advocate for me. She convinced the nurse to let me try turning over and doing some bearing down to a squat position. This helped me find the 'sweet spot' for pushing and some progress was made.

Unfortunately there was always this sense of urgency about the situation. Outside the OR room were about 13 staff waiting to 'save me' from myself and deliver my baby for me. Or to be fair, to whisk in and save lives if an emergency arose. My doula has seen too many 'failure to progress' hospital interventions and would urge me to really make each push count or I might lose my birth.

Was that really true? I'm not sure. My doc said it wasn't. He told me after that every time he wanted to swoop in and help me along, he'd leave the room and go do something else. He even delivered another baby during that time. All I know is that my husband brought his camera and there are an awful lot of pictures of men with their arms folded, standing around.

But eventually the nurse got impatient and brought up the ol' knees in ears thing again. Instead, my doula and my husband each supported a leg and gave me their hand. I was to pull on their hands, bearing the energy down and out. They provided tension against my legs and feet that made the pushes work. The other thing I finally surrendered to was the one thing that had been bothering me all along. I had read so often in natural birth advice to never hold your breath while pushing. You should 'breathe the baby out'. Also that my body would push for me if I would just let it.

Only when I started doing the work of pushing and forcing a third push off of my two contractions while holding my breath and then taking a quick one in between, did the baby descend more efficiently. The doctor came in to catch the baby. His idea of perineal support was inserting his finger in the opening and swooping it around the baby's head. Ouch, now that hurt! I wanted him to stop so badly I pushed that much harder to just get his finger out from an already stretched area. Thus Baby A, Sean Edward, was born at 6 lbs 2 oz, 19 inches. His Apgar was 8 then 9 at 7:13 P.M. after 2 hours of pushing.

Once Sean was out, they put him on my chest while the entourage came pouring into the room. I was told to push NOW! I said, but I don't have any contractions yet. They didn't care. Push now! I firmly kept my hand pressing in the new cavity where Baby A had been while my doula held her hand firmly at the base so we could keep Baby B in exactly the position he had been in. If he went transverse, everything would go south to a C-section for me. Breech or vertex-no problem I could do that. So I summoned some extra determination and just bore down. Seth Thomas was easily born 7 minutes after his brother; it was made especially easy by the fact he was a whole pound smaller, 4 lb 15 oz! His Apgar was 8 then 9.

The thing that surprised me was how alert I was during the whole thing. While I did mentally shut out the extra people in the room, I never went away to "Labor land" or even lost my ability to make calculated decisions. I'm glad because I had so many odds not in my favor allowing a twin birth to simply be a normal birth. Luckily my homework and choices for providers and a little luck from a couple of baby boys who politely kept their arms tucked in and positions ideal all came together to create the best birth I could ask for in a hospital setting with twins.

Funny last note; there was a surreal thing that happened while I was being wheeled out of the OR back to the labor and delivery room. Right outside the door was an entire Lamaze class. Here I am, a sight after birthing, holding my two vernex covered babies in my arms, and there's all these strangers staring at me. I was told it was a class; I instantly went into teacher mode and proclaimed, "A twin birth vaginally with no meds! You can do it! It's totally possible!" Everyone laughed. My husband heard the next day that another lady who birthed that evening after me used me for inspiration to get her through.

Ayla

My birth stories are brief and not too exciting, but hopefully some encouragement for those looking for "proof" that pain-free natural child births actually do exist.

With Ayla, my water broke around 3:00 a.m. at home. I phoned my doctor to see if she'd like me to come in because I wasn't having contractions yet - but due to a history of very fast labors, she wanted me near her so we took off. I arrived at my hospital which is a very natural childbirth friendly facility around 3:30 a.m. I presented my birth plan - which basically stated I'm a no-intervention-whatsoever mama and will holler when I am ready to push - and got "ready" to have my daughter. No one bothered me with IVs or internal exams or anything, and they put us right next to the kitchen so I could have my unlimited coffee and snacks.

Mild contractions began around 5:00 a.m., and got slightly stronger by 5:30 a.m. I would relate the pain of the contractions to be like a painful bowel movement - not really "pain", per se - more discomfort until the passing. At 5:45 a.m. I told my doc I was ready to push... three pushes, five minutes later, our beautiful perfect daughter was born. At 8 lbs 5.6 oz she is a perfect size, no coning of the head, nothing. We were released to go home at 10:30 a.m. - *less than 5 hours after she was born*. Not having interventions made recovery so smooth and easy, both mama and baby were ready to boogie right away!

I used basic "hypno" methods even though I didn't take any formal classes with any of my children. All of their births were similar. I used a mind-over-matter approach to pain management, being fully aware that my body is capable of natural childbirth with no medical intervention, aware of every sensation my body had, and aware that I could control my discomfort with the power of persuasion. I hope I can encourage someone else to realize the horror stories don't have to be made true. Simply by you reading this book, it tells me that you are seeking out information to empower yourself and take control of your own childbirth - and you'll do great!

Oh, by the way, we were the first baby of 2008 in our hospital, and got a boatload of goodies!

Charles Henry

Not in the Red Tent

One of my favorite books is *The Red Tent* by Anita Diamant. It's the story of the four wives of Jacob (of Abraham, Isaac, and Jacob Fame in the Bible): Rachel, Leah, Zilpah, and Bilhah, and the one daughter, Dinah. The women go to the Red Tent to give birth, have their menses, and bond with each other.

For my first two births, I had a need to go to the "Red Tent"; to be surrounded and supported by women. I was grateful to my husband for his presence, but also felt the need for the additional aid of women who knew what I was going through and could give me the verbal support I needed.

To that end, for my third birth, I made sure women surrounded me. I asked my mom to come and invited two friends, one who is interested in birth and another who wants to become a midwife. I was especially looking forward to having my mom there to tell me what a good job I was doing and to suggest different positions to labor in. I had sent her a copy of Janet Balaska's *Active Birth* and I read it myself during this pregnancy. My daughter, who is seven, also wanted to be there. I had attended the births of two of my siblings and felt that I benefited immensely from those experiences. Watching my mom give birth naturally gave me the courage to have natural births myself.

I started having contractions Friday night and could not sleep at all for watching the minutes tick by and trying to write down the contractions in the dark. As near as I could tell, they were ten to twenty minutes apart. The next morning we went to the hospital around 10:00 a.m. The doctor checked me and said I was about a 3 or a 4. "You're not in active labor yet," she told us, "Go for a walk. If you squat during the contractions, you will probably go faster."

I live in rural Alaska, and even though we have a hospital, it is more like a clinic. They only deliver low risk pregnancies, as there is no NICU, no operating room, no epidurals, and no c-sections. If it looks like there is going to be a problem, they med-evacuate you to Anchorage. After weighing all my options, I felt like my chances of having a good birth were to stay in my hometown. Rather than go to Anchorage a month before the birth and figure out what my older two children would do about school and how to get my husband to the birth in time.

I liked being told to be active which was very different from my first birth, where I stayed in a bed the whole time. So we all trekked outside. It was a cool day, and we had to drive home to get jackets and to town to buy oranges and check the mail. We got back to the hospital around 11:00 a.m. and walked for about an hour. Every time I had a contraction, my husband would support me while I squatted for about thirty seconds. For the other thirty seconds of the contraction, I turned around and hugged him while he stroked my back and breathed softly in my ear.

By noon, I couldn't walk any longer. When the doctor checked me, she said, "Well…" and I thought she was going to say something benign like, "You're making progress…" but she said, "You're at an 8 or a 9!" I had told myself that I just had to make it to 5 cm and then I could use the tub. I had given birth to my daughter in the bathtub and it was an amazing experience. The hospital personnel here were not comfortable having a water birth (and the bathtub was a little small), but people often use it to labor in. I got in the Jacuzzi bathtub for about fifteen minutes and it was great. Although the contractions were just as strong,

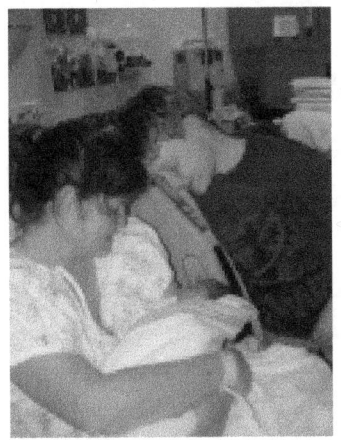

the water pulsing gave me something else to focus on.

For all three births, I've found that my body does fine right up until the pushing part and then it gets hard. This birth was no different. I could feel the baby moving down the birth canal. I got out of the bathtub and into a squatting position on the bed. My husband supported me on one side and the nurse on the other. I pushed a couple of times and the doctor said she could see the baby crowning. I thought to myself, "He's only crowning…I'm never going to get his whole head out!" It seemed like I had a long ways to go. I asked the doctor if I could push in between contractions because then I had more control and could push more slowly. She said that was fine. Then she told me the baby was almost there—maybe just two more inches to go. That felt like a long ways to me. But another contraction came, and there he was! I looked down to watch as Charles slid out. Indescribable.

My daughter watched the whole thing from the doctor's elbow. The doctor later said she wasn't sure who was going to deliver the baby—my daughter or her—as my daughter stood there intently throughout the whole thing.

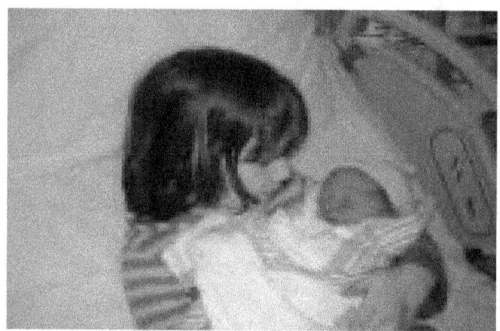

Giving birth at this rural hospital was a great experience. I was the only one giving birth at the time. I was able to try out a variety of positions while laboring. The hospital honored all of my wishes. The doctor put Charles up on my belly immediately following his birth. She did not cut the cord right away. She did not give me a shot of pitocin after the birth to help the placenta come. In fact, the doctor was surprised at how little I bled. No eye drops, no vitamin K, no PKU (we came in a week later after my milk came in to have that test). And no making me feel guilty for the decisions I had made.

But the best part of the experience was how close it made me feel to my husband. I was so grateful for his solidness throughout it all. Knowing my mom would be there helped me feel good about my decision to stay in my hometown. She came out a week early and we had a great time going for walks and organizing. But for the labor itself, I found myself relying most on my husband. It was an intimate experience that helped us draw closer together. Sometimes the "Red Tent" is needed, but for this birth I was grateful for the sweat lodge.

Mom	: Kristin
Dad	: Ben
City State	: Alaska
Age at birth	: 37
Birth	: Third
Baby's name	: Charles Henry

Birth Center Births

Alex and Andre

It was October 31st and I was rushing to get the rest of my belongings out of my apartment and into storage. I was pregnant with twins and had just lost my job that day because I had been on bed rest for too long. So much for bed rest! Because of the financial mess, we were forced to break our lease and move in with family. My boyfriend and I stayed up until 7:00 a.m. (November 1st) before we finally decided to call it a night!

Around 11:45 a.m. we woke up and as soon as I sat down in the dining room my water broke! By 12:30 p.m. we were over at my mother-in-law's house and by 1:00 p.m. I had my first contraction. Around 2:00 p.m. I had my boyfriend drive me to my mother's house to meet up with my sister, who is studying to be a midwife. My mom was at work so we had to wait for her to get home. The midwife told me to be at the birthing center by 3:30 p.m. so I knew we had time. It was almost 3:30 p.m. when we all got there. I was dilated to a 7 and fully effaced when I arrived and by 4:30 p.m. I had started pushing. Alex was born at 5:00 p.m. but their placenta (which started out as two but fused into one late in the pregnancy) started coming out before I could deliver Andre. The midwife gently took Andre's feet and, as I pushed, she pulled him out. Andre was born at 5:43p.m. Alex was 6lbs 9oz and Andre was 6lbs 8oz, and both measured 19 inches. They were born right at 37 weeks, which is considered full term for twins! Around 9:30 p.m. the midwife gave me a dose of Tylenol. By 11:30 p.m.

the twins and I arrived at my mother-in-law's house and went to bed!

Mommy	:April Castner
City State	:Dallas Tx.
Age at birth	:21
Birth	:First and Second
Baby's name	:Alexander Joel
Baby's Height	:19 inches
Baby's weight	:6lbs 9oz
Baby's name	:Andre Ezekiel
Baby's Height	:19 inches
Baby's weight	:6lbs 8oz

Nicholas Raymond

June 5th, at 5:00 a.m. on the dot, I woke up because of a really painful contraction. Just a week earlier I had false labor, so I just blew it off until 7:00 a.m. when they started getting closer together. I called my sister and she called my mom. Around 8:00 a.m. I called my midwife and she said to meet her at the birthing center at 10:00 a.m. I called a neighbor to come help get my twin boys to daycare then called another friend to drive me to the birthing center.

I got to the birthing center at 9:40 a.m., the midwife and her assistant got there at 9:50 a.m. I went to the bathroom, and then on the way back to the bed my water broke. The midwife started the water for the tub, then checked me and said I was dilated to a 10. She told me I wouldn't make it to the tub. My family wasn't even there yet. I lay down in the bed and pushed for 3 minutes. Nicholas Raymond was born at 10:05 a.m. My mom walked in 3 minutes after Nick was born and my sister never even got to leave her house! Four hours after delivering I was allowed to go home!

Mom	: April Castner
Age at birth	: 23
Birth	: Third
Baby's Name	: Nicholas Raymond
Baby's Height	: 21 3/4 Inches
Baby's weight	: 8 lbs 5 oz

Homebirths

Alejandro David de los Angeles

We were having a really stressful day. It was also ridiculously hot and it was the baby's due date. Bleh, no fun. After taking a long walk of errands around the city I somehow became convinced that the only thing that would make me feel better was to spend the night away from our home (where we had a lot of people around) somewhere that had air conditioning. We booked a room at a bed and breakfast.

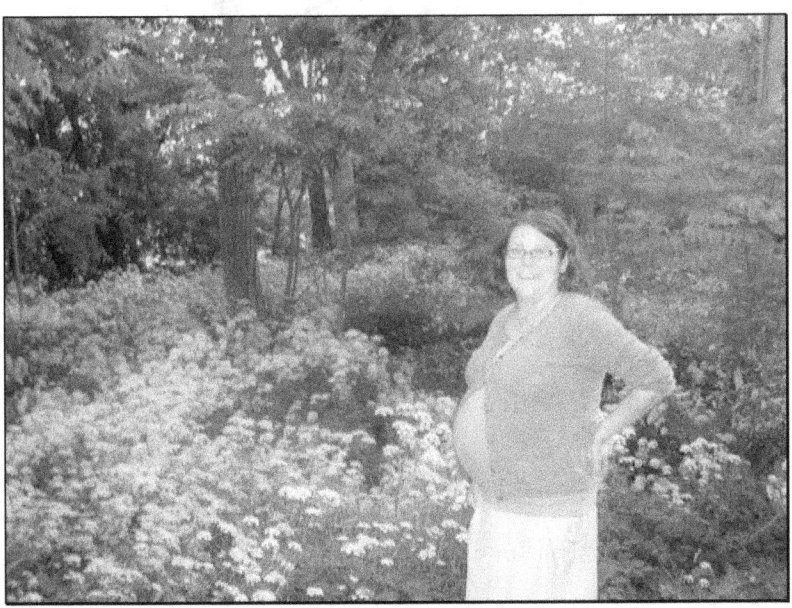

After making a nice dinner to go with us, we walked half an hour to the B&B, checked in and got settled. I felt totally relaxed. More relaxed then I had been in days. And the air conditioning, oh man!

We ate dinner and laid around in our room for about two hours. Jaime then went upstairs to pay the owner. When he was gone I felt a rush of liquid. Could my water be breaking? When he came back down to our room I had a completely stunned look on my face. "What's wrong?" Jamie asked. "My water just broke!" I exclaimed. This was at 8:00 p.m. We packed up our stuff, talked to the owner (who we ended up paying half of the fee to.) and called a cab. In the cab we joked with the driver about the weather without telling him I was in early labor.

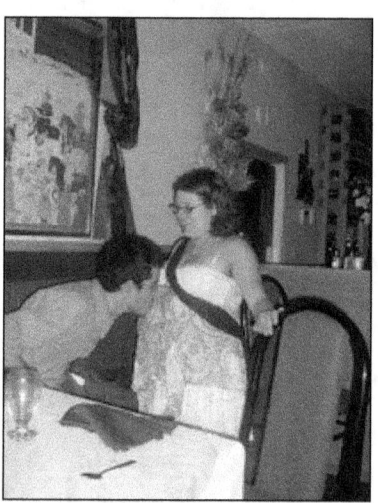

We live in an intentional community and share a house with four other people. However, no one was there when we got home. We peaked out into the backyard where a bunch of the other members of our community (a three house complex) were. We told them that I was in labor and everyone congratulated us.

Two of our housemates showed up and we talked about what they could do. I called the midwife around 8:30 p.m. and she told me to call her when the contractions were more intense. On the phone with her I had my first contraction. Whoa, it was pretty strong. But I trust my body and just went with it.

After about an hour of hanging out with our housemates, Jaime and I went up to our room to prepare the bed and birth room. My contractions were low and painful but I could still talk and walk. They kept getting more and more painful. I was thinking I would be able to sleep in early labor and kept trying to lie down, but lying down was unbearable. The only thing that helped was swiveling my hips while leaning against our dresser. So that's what I did. I was always able to talk through the contractions. Jaime and I kept repeating, "Each contraction is bringing our baby one step closer to us. My body knows what to do. I am doing this."

The contractions were coming really close together, but we weren't timing because we still thought I was in early labor. But then there was no pause in between. I remember begging the baby to wait for five minutes and to let me have a little break. This whole time I continued to talk and walk through the contractions. Jaime convinced me to call the midwife again. I had three contractions on the phone with her and she decided to come over thinking I was maybe 6 or 7 centimeters dilated.

While we waited for her we asked my housemates to set up the pool because I had decided that hot water would help. The midwife had said not to go in the bath because my water had broken but at this point I was

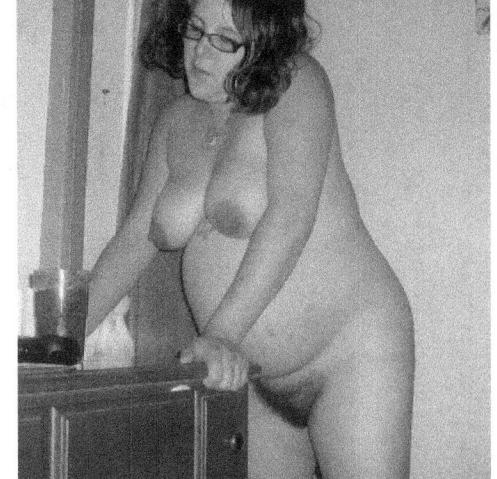

just yelling, "I want to go in the bath! I want the midwife to come! I want to go in the bath!"

Jaime convinced me to go in the shower while we waited for the midwife. I had no pauses between contractions they were just coming one on top of the other. Jaime held me up while I danced around the shower, chanting, "Every contraction brings our baby one step closer to our arms".

The midwife arrived and I immediately felt calmer. She took one look at me and suggested I take some rescue remedy, which I did. She helped me breathe through two more fast contractions and then examined my cervix.

Her: You're almost dilated.

Me: When you say almost dilated do you mean like 8 or 9 centimeters?

Her: No I mean anterior lip only. You're about to have your baby!

The midwife sprung into action, calling our second midwife and mobilizing our housemates to boil water, make juice and do other things. Apparently, I had been in transition in the shower, although still able to talk during contractions and hold my cup to drink water or juice in between them. Once I knew that this was as intense as it was going to be I relaxed completely. While the midwife was organizing everyone, I tried to go pee. After being on the toilet for a minute I started to have a contraction so stood up. I had an unbearable urge to push. So I pushed while Jaime held me up. I went back into our room, told the midwife I was ready to push. Pushing was awesome compared to the crazy fast contractions

I had been having. I got a three or four minute break in between the contractions. Pushing felt really satisfying.

Our second midwife arrived and we talked and joked between pushes. Then I felt his head. One midwife offered me a birthing stool and Jaime sat behind me to hold my hands. I could feel the baby's head in my birth canal. I pushed and pushed, taking full advantage of the rests in between. I was sounding my baby out with ferocious, beast like moans!

Our whole community was waiting outside the door to our bedroom. As the baby descended and started to push on my perineum I remember starting to sing "Ring of Fire" in my head. I also was present enough in my mind to tell Jaime how sad I felt for women who have to lie down while birthing. As well as instructing him on the proper way to wipe a woman's bottom.

Alejandro was born after four hours of intense labor, with only a half-hour of

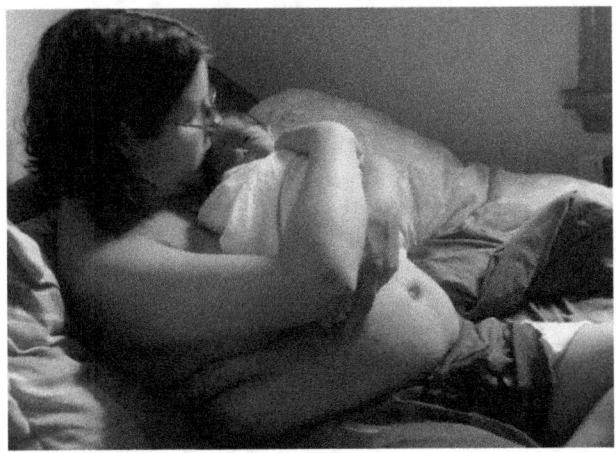

pushing. I pushed maybe 10-15 times and he came all out in one push! The midwives wrote on my chart that I was making jokes between pushing contractions...they said I was one of the quickest first births they've had. My housemate made a joke that because I read fast and walk fast than of course I would birth fast!

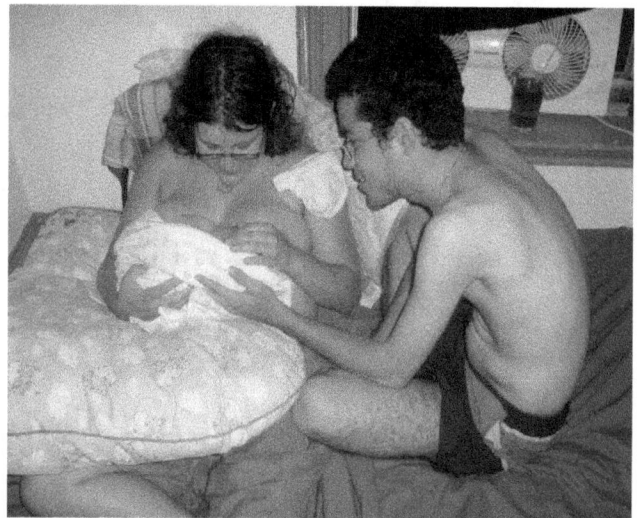

My partner was the most amazing support during the labor...I thought I would want a woman around but Jaime is extremely caring and gentle, perfect for what I needed.

Alejandro was 6 lbs 4 oz and perfectly healthy. We're getting to know him. I wouldn't have changed a thing about his labor. It was perfect! Alejandro David de los Angeles entered this world June 27 2007 at 1:04AM. He is his father's 23rd birthday gift!

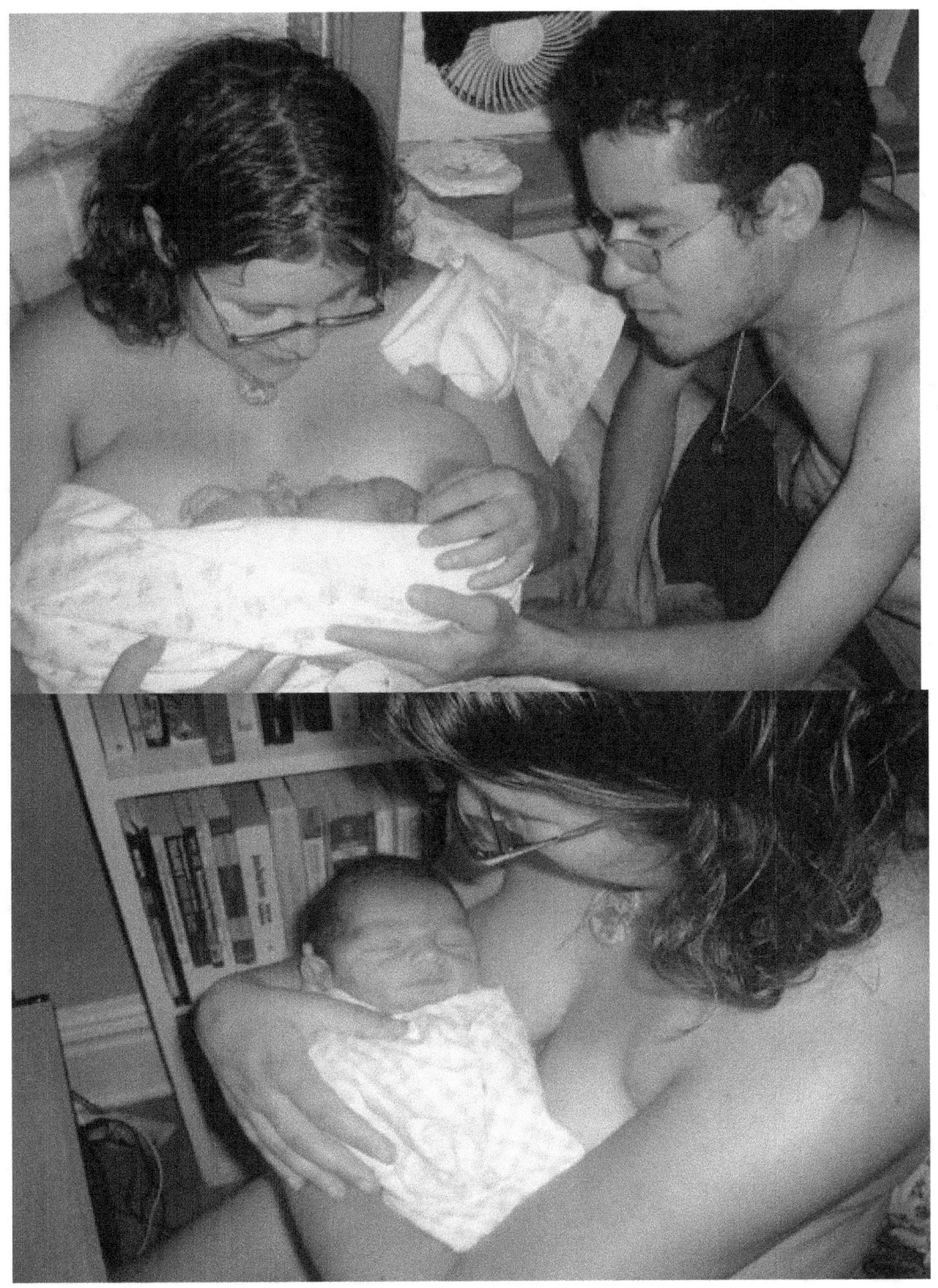

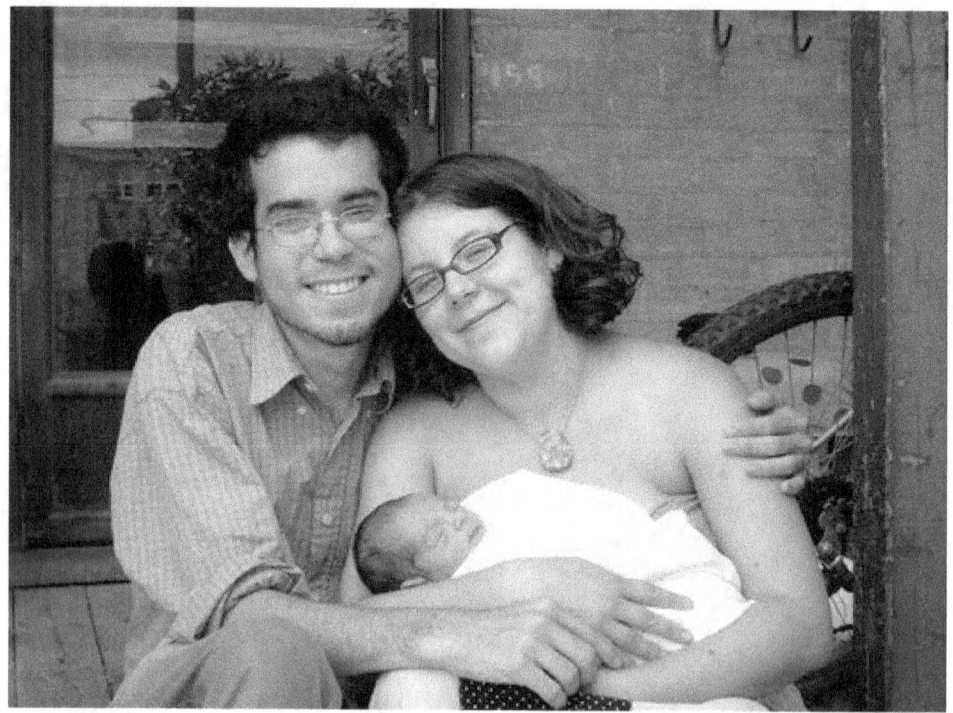

Mommy	:Elsa
Daddy	:Jamie
City State	:Petersborough, ON Canada
Age at birth	:24
Birth	:1
Baby's Name	:Alejandro David de los Angeles
Baby's Weight	:6lbs 5oz

Carson Moss

We spent the day on the 28th of October getting the rest of the pool supplies together. We had to go to the hardware store for an adapter for the tub. We came home and put the pool in the bedroom on top of blankets and a tarp. We went to a Halloween/birthday/costume party in the afternoon. I ate a ton of food, which included healthy and not so healthy stuff like cake, soda and chips. That night we watched a movie and I decided that I was going to go to bed around 11:45 p.m. because I was feeling a little achy in my back. I was afraid that I might go into labor either over night or the next morning and I didn't want to be tired. I lay down with my sleeping daughter and about twenty minutes later, I started to feel like I was having rushes. I had been having practice rushes for about two months on and off but these felt different. I got up and told Bryce that I thought maybe this was it. He hooked up the hose for the pool and we moved Leigh to the spare bedroom to sleep.

I was having trouble trying to figure out how far apart the rushes were because they got pretty intense right away. I was leaning over the side of the tub while we were filling it so I could breathe through them. Somehow, I was able to determine that they were about 1-2 minutes apart but they were not a minute long. I had Bryce get my phone and I called Wendi my midwife she said, "Do you think you need me to come now?" And I said "pretty soon". I then had Bryce call my doula, Michelle. I had called them at 1:36 a.m.

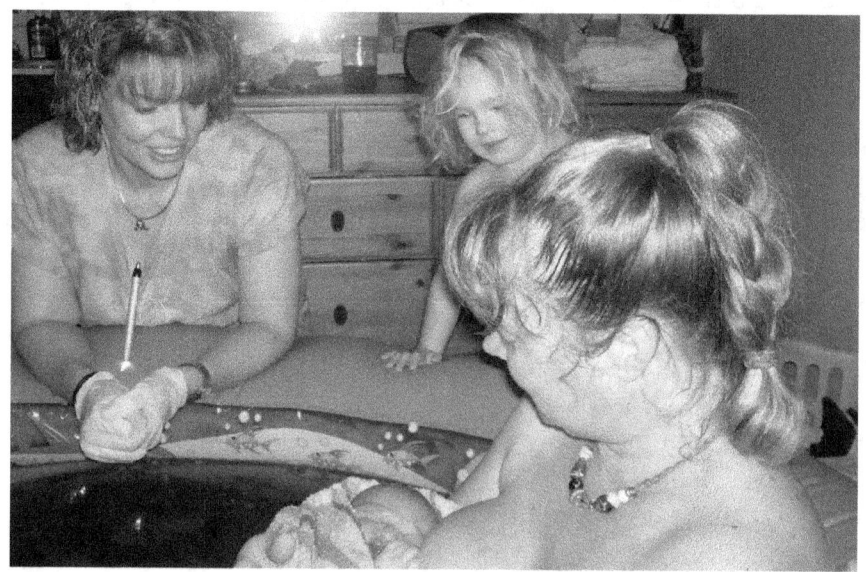

I got into the pool, which was still filling and I felt much better. The rushes were coming right on top of each other now. I got out of the pool to go to the bathroom. Wendi, Michelle and the other midwife, Stephanie all arrived. I remember thinking that our dog barking was pissing me off and I may have said, "Shut the fucking dog up!" I know I thought it! I wanted to get back in the pool after using the bathroom but I was afraid that I would slow down my labor. I asked Wendi about it and she said that she didn't think I needed to worry about it. So I got in and Wendi had brought the birth stool because I had said I wanted to try it but after a very quick second on that, I wanted it out of the pool.

Being on my hands and knees was the most comfortable position. After only a couple more contractions, I needed to push. With one big push, I felt a strong pressure and a popping. I thought at first that was his head. Wendi told me that my water had broken. With the next contraction, I pushed his head almost out and then one more and he was out. He was born with his hand aside his head, just like Leigh had been. It was 2:48 a.m., less than 3 hours from my first rush. Bryce caught him and held him until I turned around and sat down and saw that it was a boy! He was 8 lbs 2 oz and 20 inches long. We wrapped him in a towel and I held him to me for a few minutes until I birthed the placenta. Part of the placenta was retained but worked its way out after a few days.

We named our son Carson after Bryce's granddad Jack Carr who passed away this spring. His middle name, Moss, means 'from the water' so we thought that was fitting since he was born in the water.

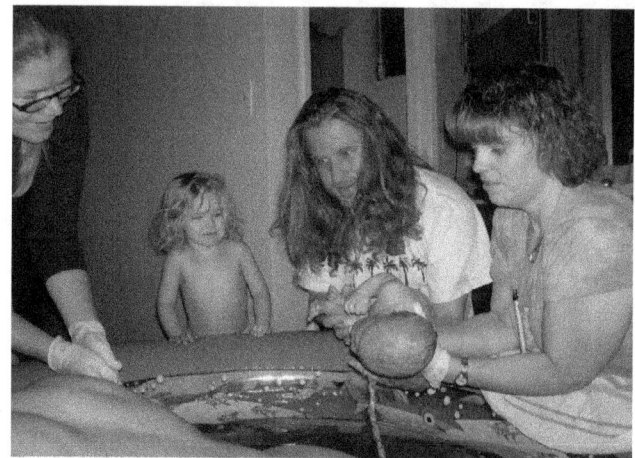
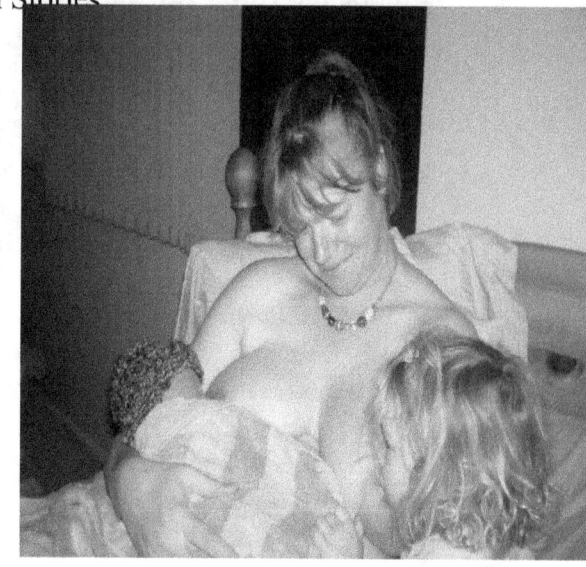
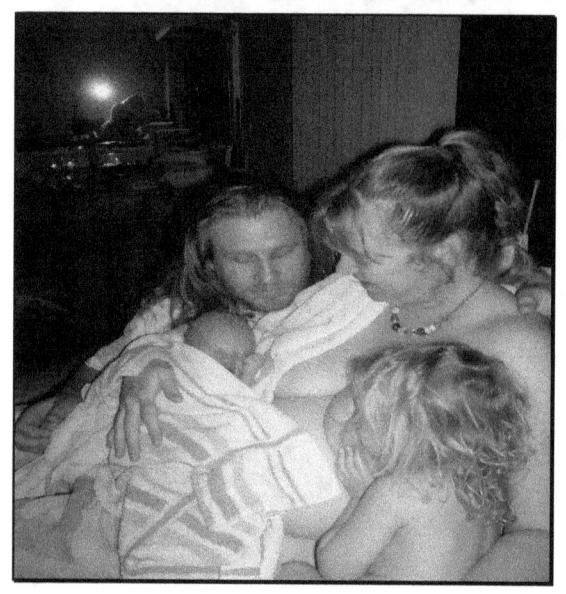
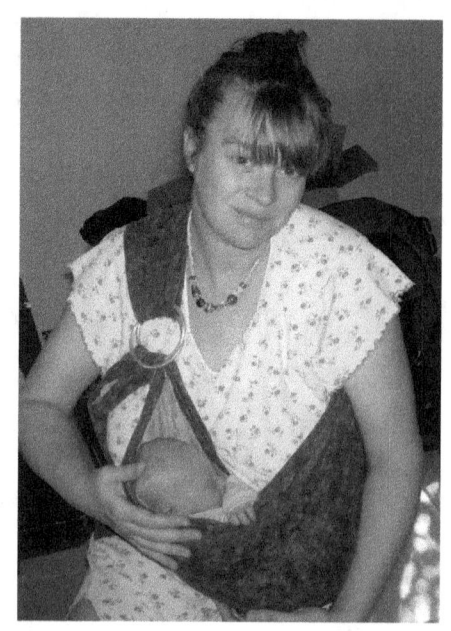

Mom	: Michelle
Dad	: Bryce
State	: AZ
Age at birth	: 37
Birth	: Second
Baby's Name	: Carson Moss
Baby's Height	: 20.5"
Baby's Weight	: 8lb 2oz

The Birth of Gabriel Ryan Stille

Perfect. That is the only word I can think of to describe my pregnancy and birth. Ryan and I got married December 18, 2005, and by the beginning of January, I wanted to be pregnant. The only problem was that I wasn't scheduled to graduate until May 2007, a year and a half away. I started reading books, most of which came from my mom, and charting my cycles to prepare for (and to prevent for the time being) pregnancy. Ryan and I had many conversations about when we would try to get pregnant. I was a little apprehensive about being pregnant and in school full time simultaneously, but I eventually decided that I trusted my body to grow a baby and allow me to continue my daily life at the same time. On a road trip in mid August of 2006, Ryan and I finally decided when we would try to conceive: my cycle closest to the beginning of October. That way, the baby would be born about two months after graduation. I think we picked out Gabe's name during that trip, too. We never fully settled on a girl's name.

I kind of assumed I would have a homebirth because well, why not? I looked into my hospital and birthing center options just to make sure I did in fact know what I wanted. I discovered that the birth I wanted was not possible in a hospital where we live and the only birthing center in the state was three hours away. When I began to search for homebirth midwives, I was completely shocked to discover that homebirth midwives cannot legally practice in Georgia. As I talked to my mom, a huge advocate of homebirth, and read more about childbirth in America, I decided the only birth I would have would be a homebirth. The backwards Georgia law was no deterrent for me, although it saddened me to learn of the state's ignorance surrounding pregnancy and childbirth.

Fast forward to October 12: I'm pregnant! My period wasn't even due for about four more days, but I just could not wait to take the test. I immediately began seeking midwife recommendations. I was already familiar with the midwives in the area, but had not spoken to any. By the time I was six weeks pregnant we had chosen a midwife. We would have to pay completely out of pocket of course because of the law.

I loved being pregnant. My pregnancy never interfered with school, although I wasn't able to keep up with the workouts I was used to. Before I was even showing, my mom announced that she thought the baby was a boy. As soon as I started showing, everyone who saw me either asked if the baby was a boy or they told me the baby was a boy. I was told that carrying low means it's a boy and I was apparently carrying low. My mom even bought blue baby clothes. This might have something to do with why we never settled on a girl's name.

Since it was my first pregnancy and pregnancy, like all of life, can be rather unpredictable, I really wanted to have a doctor I could go to should a complication arise during pregnancy or birth. However, most doctors will not see women who are planning homebirths. My midwife referred me to a homebirth friendly doctor two hours away. We went to this doctor to get the standard prenatal blood work and Pap smear done, but the doctor retired before my pregnancy ended.

During my second trimester, my midwife established a relationship with an obstetrician who was new to the area and had come from a state where midwives practice legally. He provided medical back up for homebirthers when he practiced there. He was much closer and had hospital privileges at the hospital we would want to go to in the event of a transfer. Shortly after our first appointment with him, my midwife informed me that he would no longer provide back-up care for homebirthers because of some issue with his malpractice insurance company. We were disappointed, but decided to go to our next scheduled appointment with him unless he formally dismissed us from his care.

At our next appointment, he brought up the topic. I gave him my sad face and played dumb. I was 33 weeks pregnant by this time. The topic kind of dwindled away after he mentioned that I would need to sign some form, and I gave him the results of my two-hour glucose test. He agreed that this was an accurate way of determining glucose tolerance and did not request that I take the standard glucose tolerance test with glucola. We made another appointment and left. We did not openly mention homebirth to our obstetrician anymore, but at our subsequent appointments, he would ask questions like, "Have you had any internal exams lately?" indicating that he was in no way unclear of our plans to give birth at home.

I was very happy with the prenatal care I received from him. His nurse commented a few times that she wished all their pregnant moms were as healthy and calm as me. My midwife would probably not describe me as calm since I tend to get alarmed if anything about me is anywhere near the border of what is considered normal, although my temperament was generally calmer during pregnancy than it was before. Most of the time, I felt like everything was right in my world.

My obstetrician did the same things my midwife did: check my blood pressure, weight, and urine and palpate my belly. He never asked to do ultrasound, internal exams, or any other kind of testing. He did the group B step test because I wanted it done, although my midwife could have done it. I did finally get a letter formally dismissing me from his care when I was 37 weeks, but I continued to see him. At my 38-week appointment, I signed a form stating that I understand that my obstetrician "does not participate in planned homebirths in any capacity." At my 39-week appointment, he told me to go ahead and make a 40-week appointment but he didn't expect to see me next week. I did have to call and cancel that 40-week appointment when Gabriel was born on June 23, 2007 at 39 weeks and 6 days.

Before I got pregnant and even in early pregnancy, I was a bit scared of giving birth, but by my third trimester, I had no fear at all. I probably watched about twenty birth videos since my midwife loaned me two at each prenatal visit, and I can't imagine anything preparing me better than that. We never got around to taking childbirth classes and for some reason; I didn't feel particularly compelled to do so. But really, I wasn't prepared at all and that was a good thing. I never imagined what it might actually *feel* like to give birth, and I'm glad I didn't know. Giving birth was the most wonderful experience of my life, but I wouldn't have wanted to know what it would feel like beforehand.

I felt like I was in labor my whole last month of pregnancy. By 36 weeks, the baby had "dropped," requiring that I get up to use the restroom four or more times a night instead of one or two. I was still working on campus with Ryan surveying fire hydrants four hours a day at this time. I think I found all the bathrooms on campus.

On Wednesday, Ryan and I hung out at home, went swimming, and then went to our favorite restaurant. That night, my mucous plug started to come out. I was also having contractions and I couldn't sleep. Eventually, Ryan woke up and I had to tell him what was going on. He was very excited, but I told him not to get too excited just yet because it could still be a few days. My mucous plug finished coming out about 24 hours later. My contractions felt "different" on Thursday morning, maybe just stronger. I told my mom this and she started her two-week vacation on Thursday afternoon, despite me telling her that it could still be a while. Friday morning, my contractions felt "different" again. They didn't feel like menstrual cramps anymore. They would come at regular intervals, ten to twenty minutes apart, for an hour or two at a time and then go away for thirty minutes to an hour.

I had been sitting at home for two days and it was driving me crazy. My contractions got closer together when I walked, so I avoided going anywhere for the practical reason that I had to stop walking every few minutes, annoying both myself and Ryan and probably alarming anyone who happened to see me. The whole time I had been pregnant and showing, people made comments everywhere I went, except at school, where other students looked at me like they were scared of me. My mom came over for dinner and then we went for a short walk. We returned from our walk at 9:00 p.m. and my contractions starting coming every 5-10 minutes. My mom asked if she should stay the night "just in case," but I told her no as I had been having contractions for days and for her to not get her hopes up.

My mom went home and Ryan and I went to bed to read together like we do every night. My contractions continued and I didn't want to read anymore. We turned out the light to go to sleep. That lasted about ten minutes. I got up and walked around, leaning on my dresser during contractions. Ryan was timing them. I was starting to think we might have a baby soon. The contractions were coming every four to seven minutes. At about 10:15 pm, I said maybe we should call the midwife to let her know what's going on before it gets too late. I talked to her for about twenty minutes and she told me to call back when the contractions were under five minutes apart for an hour. As soon as I got off the phone, my contractions started coming every three to four minutes and got stronger. Standing got to be uncomfortable so I sat on my exercise ball. Ryan called my mom to come over. I stopped looking at the clock at this point. I read somewhere that it's discouraging to look at the clock during labor. I did keep asking Ryan how long it had been since I got off the phone with the midwife because I wanted to know when we could call back.

I think somewhere around 11:30 p.m., I told Ryan to call the midwife and I don't want to talk, I'm busy. Ryan called and then asked me, "Do you want them to come now?" "Yes!" I replied. I started feeling nauseous and constantly hot than cold. Ryan had already set up the living room by this time. The pool was ready to be filled up and the old futon was on the floor. I really wanted my midwife to get there so I could get in the pool. I had no idea how far along I was. The exercise ball became uncomfortable, as did standing and walking, so I went to the futon on the living room floor and plopped down on my left side with a pillow between my legs. My midwife and her apprentice arrived somewhere around midnight. My contractions kept getting stronger and it seemed like there was no break in between them. I really had to focus, making deeps sounds, to get through them. I threw up. My midwife said, "Good. That shows you're making progress." She checked my cervix and I was 8-9 cm dilated! I had no idea I was that far along. I knew that transition was supposed to be the most intense and shortest part of labor. So I didn't expect my contractions to get much stronger and I thought I would be pushing soon.

I got in the pool and the contractions slowed down. That was a much-needed break. I don't know how long the break was, but when the contractions started coming on strong again, my hips hurt no matter what position I was in. My mom and Ryan sat next to me giving me water to drink and cold wash clothes to put on my head. My midwife and her apprentice sat on the other side of the room.

An hour after my body did this very odd thing that felt like throwing up backwards. Apparently it was trying to push the baby out. My midwife came over to the poolside to check my cervix. She said I had a slight lip but it was okay to push. That was good news because my body was going to push whether I wanted it to or not. The pushing sensation was so strange and new to me that I think I involuntarily fought it for a while. My midwife suggested I try standing. I got out and did sort of a standing squat with Ryan supporting me. Immediately, I wanted to sit down, so my midwife put the birth stool underneath me. I rested on it between contractions and stood up to push. I think we did that for something like an hour. Ryan was getting tired and my hips still hurt. My midwife told me I needed to hold my breath and push during contractions. I just couldn't relax to effectively push, so I said I wanted to lie down.

I got back in the side-lying position on the futon with Ryan lifting my leg during contractions. This helped a lot with the hip pain. I guess I just needed all the pressure to be taken off my legs. I held my breath during contractions and my body did all the pushing. It just needed me to cooperate. The breath holding helped with the pain, too. I was kind of afraid to push the baby out, but I knew that was clearly what had to happen. Ryan told our midwife that he wanted to catch the baby. My birth summary says I pushed for two hours, so I think I pushed in the side-lying position for about an hour. Ryan cried that whole time. I only know that because I could hear him sniffling. I had my eyes shut most of the time. My mom was probably crying, too, but I wasn't paying any attention to her except to ask for cold wash clothes for my face.

Somebody, either my mom or my midwife's apprentice, kept giving me sips of water. I wasn't thinking about being thirsty. I was just thinking about my face being hot and feeling the "ring of fire" as the baby's head came out. I didn't want the baby to come too fast. I generally like to ease into things and feel moderate pain gradually rather than do things quickly and feel extreme pain all at once. When I ran cross-country in high school, I was never better than an average runner because I simply refused to push myself beyond what I felt was comfortable. I think I could have gotten the baby out faster if I had helped my body push a little more than I did, but I just wasn't willing to do that. When I go swimming and the water is cold, I usually take at least ten minutes to ease myself into the water. Maybe it's a control thing. I feel that if I do it at my own pace and I can think it through, I feel like I am in control.

I didn't know this until after the birth, but Gabe's right hand started to emerge with his head. Ryan told me that our midwife put his hand back in as soon as it started to come out. Ryan supported my perineum while his head came out. After his head was out, his body got a little stuck, so Ryan and the midwife tugged on Gabe.

Finally, we got him out! He was immediately placed on my chest. "Is it a boy or a girl?" I asked. Ryan told me that our baby is indeed a boy, Gabriel Ryan Stille. He latched on as soon as he was offered the breast (Which was as soon as the cord stopped pulsating and was cut). I was lying down and the cord was too short to nurse him while we were still connected. My midwife wanted to get the placenta out quickly because I was bleeding a little too much. I didn't get any more contractions, so I made the effort to push the placenta out. After 15 minutes, out it came. My midwife did a wonderful job of controlling the bleeding. She had me drink three glasses of an electrolyte drink, Emergen-C, afterwards. Ryan took Gabe and I went to the bathroom. Then I went to my bed and ate breakfast. After I was all fixed up and the newborn exam was finished, Ryan and Gabe joined me in bed, where we stayed for the rest of the day. Gabe weighed in at 8 lb 11 oz! I expected him to be smaller since Ryan and I were both in the 6 lb range at birth.

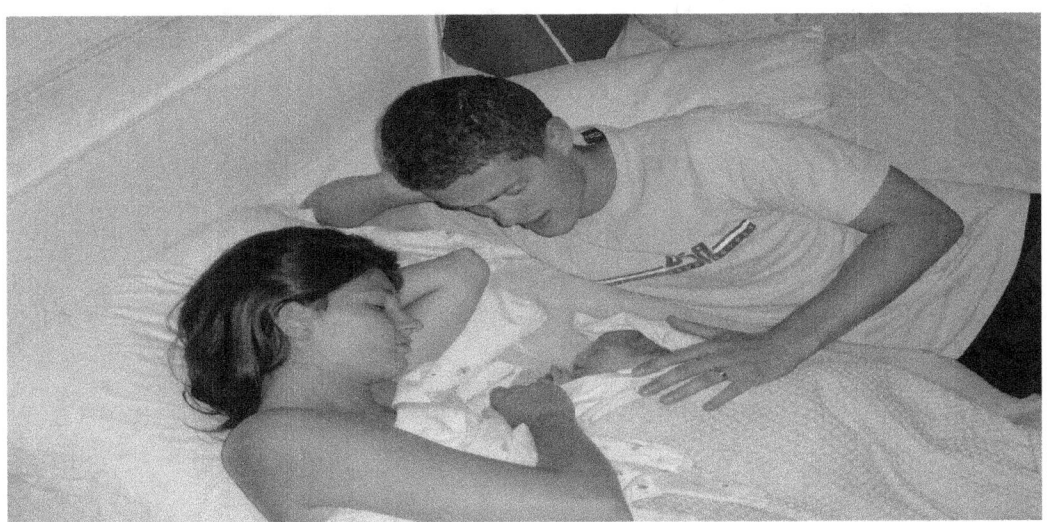

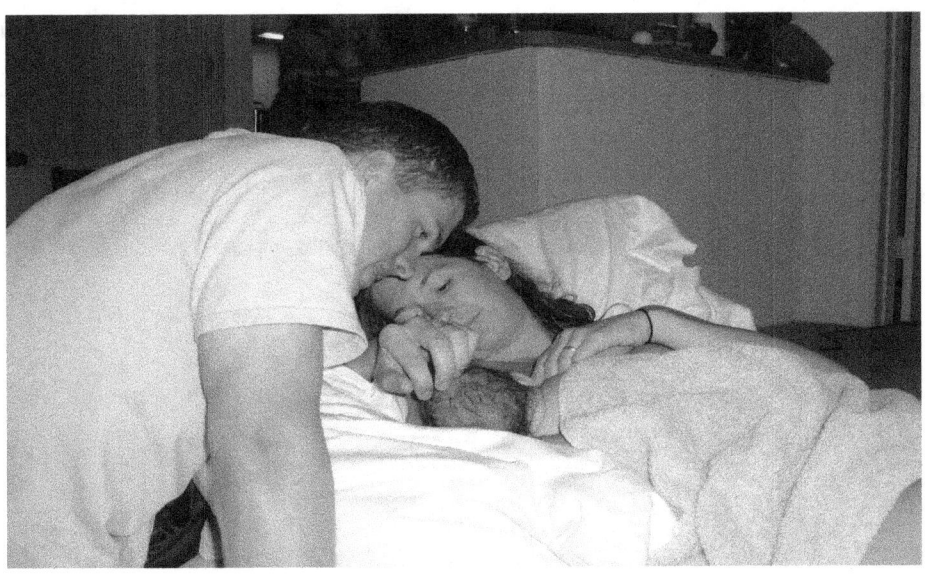

I showered the next day with Ryan's help. My mom stayed for two weeks while I recovered and she filled my freezer with yummy food. I was up and about a little bit five days after birth and took my first walk to the park with Gabe in my sling two weeks after birth. Gabe nurses constantly and I think I've lost at least 20 of the 30 pounds I gained during my pregnancy. I think my breasts have doubled in size, so I don't expect to lose any more weight, not that how much I weigh matters at all, but people like to ask me how much I gained and how much I've lost so there it is. I am looking forward to running again. Whenever that may be since my mom says I may not be able to do vigorous exercise while I'm establishing nursing.

Shortly after Gabe was born, Ryan asked me, "So you want to do that 11 more times?" since I joke about having a dozen kids. I replied that I don't want to talk about that right now. Now that it has been a little over two weeks, I can say that yes, I want to do that many more times, although I don't know how many babies I can fit into my lifetime. Hopefully, breastfeeding will fend off my fertility for a year or so. Four years is a good spacing between kids I think, but who knows. I only wish that we could live here for all of them so that I could have the same midwife. Everything was just perfect and now I have a perfect baby boy.

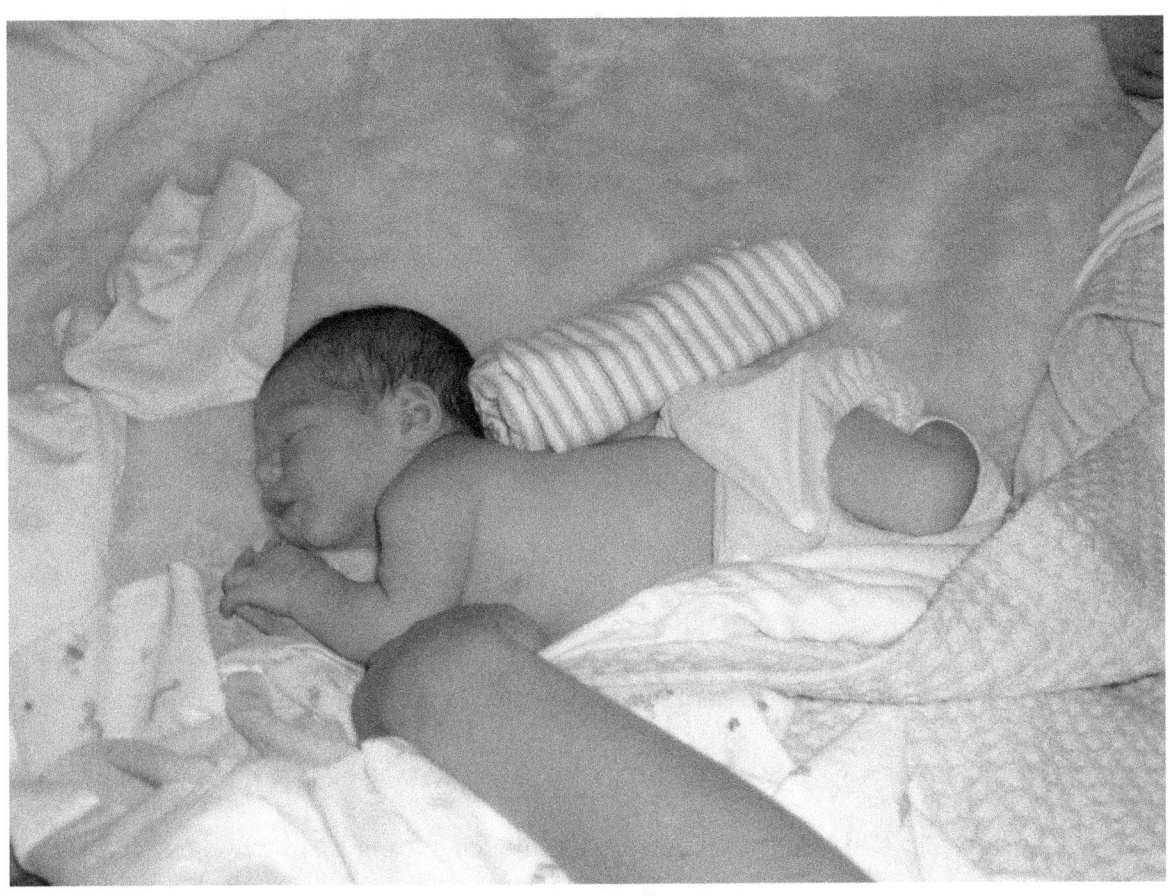

Mom	: Michelle
Dad	: Ryan
City State	: Atlanta, GA
Age at birth	:22
Birth	: First
Baby's Name	: Gabriel Ryan
Baby's Weight	: 8 lb 11 oz,
Baby's Height	:21 inches

Kaian Gregory

On Monday evening I started to get the feeling that I'd be in labor very soon. I know, I must be Nostradamus or something considering I was nine days past my estimated due date. I kept bugging my dear husband to go to the park with Riley because I knew it would be the last time we'd go out as just the three of us and I wanted some fresh air. While we were there I felt fine, a little pressure but no contractions or anything.

We came home around 7:00 p.m. and I made Kraft Mac n' cheese for dinner. I did add broccoli to give it some integrity and we had some ice cream. At about 10:15 p.m. I took Riley into her room to nurse her and started having some mild contractions. This was nothing new; I had been getting them while nursing for weeks so I didn't think much of it. At 10:40 p.m. I called Greg in to sing Riley a song and get her into her crib and I did what I always do - I bee lined it to the bathroom to pee. I had just finished my business and was sort of just sitting on the toilet waiting for the right moment to get up, when I heard and felt a strange "pop" at the top of my belly. Immediately a gush of fluid poured out of me into the toilet. I started shaking with excitement and called out to Greg that my water had broken. He was so excited he was almost dancing!

I called my midwife Kelley and she told me to try and sleep because it could be minutes or days before labor begins. I stood there as a puddle accumulated below me and I agreed to try to sleep, but I knew I'd be calling her back very soon. I took a shower and was amazed at how much smaller and lower my belly looked. After that I started to get onto all fours to try and get baby into a good position. He was head-down with his side facing out that morning when Kelley had checked. Contractions started soon after my shower and were pretty strong and surprisingly close together, about 2-3 minutes apart. We called Kelley again and again she told me to sleep, but she wasn't surprised when I called her five minutes later and said she should head over since she is an hour away.

Greg got to work setting up the birthing tub and I could feel myself starting to withdraw. The surges were extremely intense now and I was leaking fluid and was finding it very hard to change positions. I was lying on my side on the floor for a long time while waiting for the tub to get full. I told Greg to call my friend Sara, who was going to be my doula. I knew I was not going to want her to do anything for me but I still wanted her to be there since she was really excited about the birth. When Sara arrived all I wanted was for her to hold one leg up for me while I labored in that same side-lying position for a while longer.

To our surprise, the tub was filling fast with murky, brown water. There had been lots of rain earlier that week and the water had been a little cloudy, but I couldn't believe how gross the water looked. When Kelley arrived she said not to worry and that I could get into the tub anyway. I wanted to be in the water but truly had to be convinced to get up and get in because I was having so much trouble changing my position. Finally I got up the strength to get into the tub and after a few minutes in the water I did feel more comfortable. It was not the blissful experience I'd expected but it was better than my last position.

I wasn't speaking to anyone unless absolutely necessary anymore. I was way too focused on "opening up" with each contraction and the surges were so strong I was making these animal sounds with them. If someone tried to move my hair or touch my shoulder I shrugged them away - I was so not interested in being touched in any way.

One wonderful thing was that everyone there totally respected this and they were quiet and did not try to force me to answer any questions or anything like that. Really the only one I talked to at all was Kelley and that was to let her monitor the baby's heart rate, which remained perfectly strong! Also to say no thanks to Greg and Sara, who kept offering me sips of Recharge. Kelley told me later I was very polite lots of pleases and thank you. Whenever someone offered to do something for me I would respond; "I want nothing." I had no concept of what time it was. I was exhausted, sweating, and believe it or not, nodding off between contractions. I kept feeling my face hit the water and I'd wake up to another strong bolt going through my body. It's funny, but as quiet and serious as I was, I had Bob Marley in my head all night.

There definitely came a point where I said "how much longer?" and "I can't do this!" and Kelley very quietly assured me that I could and was doing it and told me how great I was doing. I felt the urge to push, or bear down, soon after getting into the tub. When I felt the need, I did it. I didn't ask if it was ok, Kelley told me to do whatever I needed to do. I never once knew how dilated I was because Kelley never checked and I was thankful for that. That urge to push came with some contractions and with others it didn't. It was so overwhelming there was no way I could deny it. I could not believe how strong my body could push down ... I kept feeling like I was pooping (gross I know but that's the only way to describe that feeling - like you're pushing with all your might).

At some point Kelley told me to feel inside and see if I could feel his head and I couldn't believe it - his head was right there! Once I told her I could feel the head she took the baby's heart rate and it had slowed down. She and Joyce, the other wonderful midwife who was there, suggested I change positions. She said the baby was still doing fine but now he was acting like a baby in labor. Before that she kept joking that he seemed totally unaffected, like he was having a great time. She said I should try and get him to move down a little quicker. She said I should get out of the tub and lay on the couch. I was in no mood to be moved. But I knew it would help the baby come out sooner so I used every bit of strength and stood up, leaning on Sara, and got my ass out of that tub. I wobbled over to the couch with a baby's head between my legs and laid down and immediately got to pushing.

Greg had gotten Riley out of bed (it was just about 6:00 a.m. now) and she was just watching the whole thing unfold. I thought she was going to be scared to see me in pain but she was surprisingly amused. If I yelled or moaned, she giggled. It was really nice to have her there to lighten the mood. Pushing itself felt great! What didn't was the "ring of fire." I was saying that I felt like I was tearing and Kelley kept saying "you're not tearing you're stretching!" I was like "Yeah right, oh well, F-it" and pushed with all my might. I don't know exactly how many pushes it took. Joyce was there with the mirror and I could see his little face. This made me want to hold him so bad so I gave it my all and out he slid! He was on my chest and crying and everyone was rallying around us taking pictures and the midwives were doing whatever it was they needed to do. He stayed attached to the cord for a good twenty-five minutes before they clamped it and Greg cut it. Kai got tens on both his Apgars and was wide-awake, just calmly looking around at everyone and taking it all in. I couldn't believe he'd come out of my vagina!

Once the placenta was out I laid down in our bed with the baby to nurse. I was sore and shaky and still in a bit of shock. Greg made me toast with peanut butter that tasted like wood so Kelley got me some yogurt and strawberries. Everyone really wanted me to eat and get some fluids but I was really not hungry. Riley was supercharged and running around like a nut while the midwives cleaned up our apartment so Kai and I had some alone time with Daddy.

It didn't really even hit me that I'd just had a VBAC for a while. I realized I hadn't thought about my scar even once during the entire birth. I felt totally strong and capable the whole time, even when I said I couldn't do it anymore I knew I was going to. Everyone around me had complete faith in me and I know that their positive presence helped to keep me calm and focused... and that's how little Kai came into this world

Mom	:Jean
Dad	:Greg
City/State	:Westport, MA
Age at birth	:27
What number birth is this?	:Second
(First was c-section due to too many hospital interventions)	
Baby's name	:Kaian Gregory
Baby's Height	:20.5"
Baby's Weight	:7 lbs 9 oz.

Matthew

I wanted to share the story of my Matthew's birth. He is my miracle and I want the world to know our story.

My husband and I had been married for nearly four years and had been trying to conceive for that entire time. After two miscarriages and millions of negative pregnancy tests, our prayers were finally answered. How were we able to conceive, you ask? You may not believe me, but it was because of my chiropractor. Through regular chiropractic adjustments and a little bit of nutritional support, my monthly cycle was finally regular (for the first time in my life). Within a few months of being regular, we were pregnant and rejoicing.

Because I am now a convert to chiropractic, I continued to visit the chiropractor throughout my pregnancy. Near the end, I was there at least once a week, if not twice. There is a technique called 'Webster' that really relieves a lot of discomfort. As well as it turns breech babies. I was receiving that as well as pelvic support.

Matthew was nearly two weeks late when labor finally started. My husband called my midwife at 2:30 in the morning to inform her of the situation. Because this was my fist baby, she advised us to try to get more sleep because we most likely had a long road ahead of us (considering most first-time moms have an average labor of 9-10 hours). Well, my contractions weren't lasting very long, only about 20-25 seconds, but they were coming one on top of another, which did not allow for sleep. They didn't really hurt; I attribute that to the regular adjustments I had been receiving. The only pain I felt was some back labor pains, and when my husband provided counter-pressure, that too was mostly relieved.

During one of my contractions, my water broke and my husband called the midwife again. She advised us that we had approximately 1-2 hours until the baby would arrive and it was time to head for the birth center. We had been packed for nearly a month, so we were on our way in no time.

Well, not five miles down the road my contractions changed and I couldn't keep from pushing. I felt the baby crowning, so my husband pulled over into the parking lot of Target and ran around to my side of the car just as the baby arrived - at 4:20 a.m. he quickly snatched him up, placed him on my chest, and covered us with a blanket. He was breathing just fine and kind of whimpering so we opted not to go to the birth center but rather to return home and have the midwife meet us there, as she was only a few miles from where we were.

The birth had happened so quickly, and we were so concerned with keeping the baby warm, that it wasn't until we were nearly back home that we even thought to check if we had a boy or a girl. Although it didn't matter to us either way, my husband was particularly excited to learn that he had a son. Back at our apartment we waited in the car for the midwife to arrive. She clamped the cord and I was able to cut it. I had already delivered the placenta, so we wrapped the baby up and made our way inside.

My total labor was just under two hours long, and I have a strong and healthy baby boy who is our little chiropractic miracle. My husband is now attending chiropractic school in hopes that he can help other people's dreams come true.

Ryan

Home Birth After two C-sections

Beautiful. There's no other way to describe it. Words fail me when I try to capture this journey any other way. I suspect that I will never stop reflecting upon and benefiting from the road I took to birthing my son. Despite four external versions (one of which was successful), moxibustion, Webster Chiropractic care, ice packs, music, breech tilts, hypnosis etc, and my little boy was breech when labor began at approximately 39 weeks.

My previous births were cesareans for transverse and breech, so, even before this pregnancy began, I had researched breech—ways to turn babies, as well as the safety of breech vaginal birth and the option of home birth. The research shows nearly equal outcomes for breech babies born by c-section and those born vaginally, and also shows that a VBAC is safer for the mother. Ultimately, I decided that I would proceed with a vaginal birth at home even if my baby was breech. It was a long process coming to that decision. I agonized, and soul-searched on top of researching the "facts". Surprisingly, once labor hit, my fears were not much of an obstacle.

I never felt like I had given birth to either of my children and absolutely hated the surgeries. Being tied down, and paralyzed from the spinal were absolutely terrifying to me and triggered the feelings of helplessness I had felt when I had been sexually abused as a child. Moreover, even after my second child was born, though overjoyed to have my son and daughter, I was devastated to not have achieved what I considered to be a rite of passage for women. I had always pictured myself giving birth naturally, medication-free to my children. I feel so many women take that opportunity for granted.

My husband, though wanting me to have the chance to fulfill my dream, was not interested in having more kids. He also admitted to being somewhat fearful of my propensity for falling in the minority risk-wise, so when he got lazy with birth control, and we got pregnant, I was ecstatic! I have a uterine division, called a septum, which is known to contribute to many pregnancy losses. Immediately upon finding out I was pregnant I began to connect with the baby and help him find a great spot to implant.

The comfort with and skill level of attending breech vaginal births were one of the first questions I asked prospective midwives. I was blessed to find a midwife who is a former ICAN leader, with over 20 years experience and comfortable and experienced with breech vaginal deliveries. I also had another midwife, her partner, in attendance. The four of us (they along with my husband, Andy, and I), had agreed to proceed with a breech home birth as long as I continued to show progress and the baby was doing well as assessed by fetal heart tones. This was based on the belief that when labor in a breech birth is not progressing, it is indicative of a problem that would necessitate a cesarean.

On Saturday, March 11, 2006, I began feeling heavy abdominal and cervical sensations. I also had the distinct feeling that my water could break at any moment. I decided that we had better get to the store to get what we needed for the birth (nothing like waiting until the last moment, but I had been so focused on the mental preparation, I nearly forgot the concrete, tangible pieces!). Thankfully, we also went to bed on the early side on the 11th as I woke up early Sunday morning (1 a.m.) lying in a puddle of amniotic fluid and vernix. I continued leaking amniotic fluid and mucous throughout early labor, which was a nuisance for which I hadn't been prepared.

I called the midwife and then tried to rest. Contractions began at about 2:00 a.m. and were about 6-8 minutes apart and very manageable. Though excited, I knew rest would be very important, so I popped in "When Harry Met Sally" (a favorite I had been meaning to watch for some time) and dozed off between contractions.

Contractions began to pick up around 9:00 a.m.—they were consistently three minutes apart and starting to get my attention, though still quite manageable. Sally, one of the midwives, came and checked me, and forgot we had agreed for me not to know how dilated I was (I was 3 cm). She left to do a postpartum visit with another client. We were thinking, "hurry, back" little did we know it would be more than a day before our son joined us.

Andy and my son Joshua (what a talented 5 year old) had finished setting up the birth tub. We called my friend to come with her daughter to help entertain our kids, as the contractions seemed to be getting stronger. I got into the birth tub, but didn't stay long, as I wasn't comfortable. Turns out that the tub was better for entertaining our kids than it was for me! I was absolutely giddy at the beginning stage of labor. I welcomed the privilege of laboring and birthing and for once was free of my obsession of time or fear of what "should" be happening. I let my body work! And it did, slower than I wanted it to, at times, but oh it did! One of my midwives, Jessica, commented later, that even at the end, I seemed to be appreciating labor.

At this point, having the kids around was a welcome distraction, and I was still able to be amongst everyone and manage the contractions (still 3 minutes apart). The worst part was actually shoulder and upper back pain that may have been from tensing up during contractions. By late afternoon, early evening, I began feeling the need to pace/circle my house during contractions (had been managing them sitting up, just pausing during my conversation). I also felt the need to carry a pan around as I was very nauseous and thought I might vomit, though I never did.

I started getting frustrated when the kids and/or their toys would get in my way while circling/pacing and was ready for everyone to leave (unfortunately, we were still a couple of hours from bedtime). So, Andy and I went upstairs to lie down and listen to the CD I had made of music that inspired and relaxed me. I treasure these moments. It was a wonderful time to connect with the man who has supported me all of these years and given me the gift of (now) three wonderful children.

The midwives checked me shortly thereafter and I was "on the edge of transition" (later they told me I was 6.5 cms and completely effaced). So, I was making progress, just a lot slower than we all thought would be the case. I hopped in the shower, and that helped immensely. Despite the nausea, I forced myself to eat, as I was worried I would run out of energy to push. I have always been one who did not function well on less than ideal amounts of sleep (and yet I have three kids, so I am getting good training), so I didn't want any other factors depleting my energy.

At several points during labor, I started shaking. The midwives said that this was likely the baby moving through my pelvis. I had to resist the thought that this was indicative of transition. At this point, I decided to listen to the Hypno-Birthing Affirmations Tape. This was very reassuring.

I was still feeling somewhat discouraged by the length of labor, though, so my wonderful husband, pulled me into our office, sat me in a recliner and began reading my Blessingway emails from my ICAN (International Cesarean Awareness Network) friends. It was just what I needed, to be reminded of all the love and strength supporting me from all over the world. We stayed in that room to labor, as I was as comfortable as one can be "on the edge of transition". We both dozed on and off as my contractions and noticeable moaning allowed. The midwives told me later, that my contractions spaced back out to 6-8 minutes apart during the night, allowing me to get some much needed rest.

My daughter, Serena, called for Daddy at 1:00 am. Andy went upstairs and fell asleep, so I was left to labor alone. After awhile, remembering that the midwives had expected a relatively short labor, I began to get discouraged that it was already over 24 hours. I decided I would feel better being near the midwives, so I went into the family room, where they were sleeping, to labor there. They must be used to sleeping with noisy women in labor, because they didn't wake up and I thought I was pretty loud! They continued to check on me hourly, which gave me comfort. My son's heart rate was consistently in the 130's, like the external cephalic version, he seemed to have no problem dealing with labor. This was of course, very reassuring.

After the kids got up and out of the house, the midwives suggested I get in the pool, but I wanted none of it. I got into the shower instead. Aiming the warm water on my belly really helped the contractions be more manageable. When Andy came back, he accompanied me on my laps around the house, which was so nice.

I had watched a video called "Birth Day", a documentary of a Mexican midwife's homebirth, and she had noted that when she was walking away from her husband, the contractions only felt like pain, but when she was walking toward him, she was reminded of their love for each other. I mentioned this to Andy, and he promptly began walking with me, as our doorways would allow. Walking up and down the stairs also served to help the baby drop down.

I tried the exercise ball, even though, previously, it hadn't been comfortable no matter what position I tried, and while there, asked the midwives how I would know when to push. I was very discouraged that I wasn't feeling the urge, even though, earlier, the midwives had implied I was completely dilated. It was especially nerve-wracking because I know how important it is to push a breech baby out quickly. Interestingly enough, although it was always a concern of mine in pregnancy, the thought of uterine rupture only occurred to me in passing when I would feel some twinges of adhesion pain. But, from the research I had done, I knew that's what it was, because they were minor, associated with movement and would pass.

We went upstairs at 12:00 p.m. I was still not feeling the urge to push, only occasional sharp, cervical pains that Jessica suggested was him kicking my cervix. The midwives checked me and told me that I could try "practice pushing" if I wanted to. While I did, Jessica pushed on my son externally to help get him more centered, as he had again drifted to an almost diagonal position. I tried various positions, hands and knees, birth stool, semi-sitting, etc. and nothing was comfortable.

Pushing was a great fear of mine, because I have always had trouble communicating to my body what I want it to do, and again, I knew it was of the utmost importance to push the breech baby out quickly. Intellectually, I know that I am a large-framed person and I doubted that head entrapment would really be an issue, but it still worried me some. At one point, my midwife, Sally said, "you aren't going to get the baby out pushing that way" (taking breaks during pushing). She didn't mean for it to, but this really played into my fears of not being able to push correctly. At this point, my wonderful husband said to me "think about the email you will get to compose to ICAN; start writing it in your head". He knew just what to say to give me hope! I told them I was worried and getting frustrated, so they suggested I shower and then rest with Andy.

The contractions were much stronger at this point. I got out, and tried some more pushing while Sally "held my uterus out of the way". I reportedly have a septate (divided) uterus. Very interesting, but in terms of my birth, it was necessary to actually hold some of my "huge" uterus out of the way, so that he could descend below it and into the birth canal. Despite these lengthy vaginal exams, my fear that previous sexual abuse triggers would be an issue was not realized.

I was still very frustrated with pushing and not feeling the urge, so Sally and Jessica suggested that Andy and I again lay down together to rest. Later, Sally told me that I always progressed when Andy and I spent time lying together. I thought this a wonderful testament to our relationship. The contractions were hard to handle lying down, but I was somehow able to doze between them. After only a few minutes, I had a monster contraction and literally jumped out of bed. When this happened, I headed straight for the bathroom, where I would usually have contractions one on top of the other. I heard Sally say to Andy in her mother tone "I thought she was resting". Both midwives were downstairs at this point. I asked him to ask her if I should push if I felt like it (and I did) and they said "sure". I reached down and felt into my vagina and felt something. Andy went and got the mirror and flashlight and sure enough, his foot was emerging! I could see the wrinkles on the sole of his feet—so exciting! I began grunting and involuntarily pushing at this point and suddenly heard the midwives rush up the stairs. The sound of their feet stomping up those stairs is one I will never forget! It was really getting exciting! I was going to do this!

The midwives, figuring I didn't want to have him on the toilet, quickly set up the birth stool and moved me from the toilet to it. By the time I stood up to move, his foot was hanging down. Just a few pushes (and about 7 minutes) later, and our little Ryan joined our family! It was absolutely amazing!!! I had been worried my body wouldn't know how to push, but it knew exactly what to do!!!

As soon as he was out, I began bleeding, and the midwives very calmly moved me to the floor. They kept asking me if I was there with them, and I was getting annoyed, and told them of course I was. I was just elated with my baby, our birth and my body and annoyed to be lying on the uncomfortable hardwood floor!

The bleeding slowed down and our baby moon could now officially begin! I remember noticing with great delight that evening that I had a baby in my arms and no painful incision across my belly! Oh, the joy! And, I had remarked to Andy that "I wish I had done this (breech vaginal birth) with Josh and Serena too", but then quickly realized that their births had to happen in order for Ryan's to happen the way it did. I never would have considered researching breech vaginal delivery and home birth if I hadn't experienced the emotional and physical pain of the cesareans (and found ICAN; can't get enough plugs in for them!).

It is amazing to me how far-reaching the impact of this beautiful birth has been. I truly feel like a different person; more at peace than I was before. I look at life with a lot more joy. I feel much more "whole" as a mom.

Mom:	:Christie
Dad:	:Andy
City/State	:Catskill NY
Age at birth	:32
Baby:	:Ryan
Birth	:Third
Baby's Height	:20.5 in
Baby's Weight	:7lbs 10 oz

Ellyse Quinn

I had my pregnancy pictures taken on Saturday September 15th at 39 weeks, 1 day. I thought I had at least another week to go since I had never delivered early. So after a busy afternoon at the mall, and a very busy week getting ready for my daycare site visit/inspection, we decided we weren't going to do anything on Saturday evening. Charlie and I did go out to Blockbuster and when we got home at about 7:00 p.m., I noticed that the contractions were feeling different from the ones that I had for the previous month. I text messaged my doula friend, Dee, at about 9:30 p.m. letting her know that she should not get excited, but contractions were about twenty minutes apart and we were going to bed. I slept for about two hours, and when I finally got out of bed at close to midnight, I thought that this was probably really "IT."

There really wasn't anything to do or get ready. The house was already clean and organized. I checked my email and tried to watch tv. Charlie was still sleeping during all of this even though I kept telling him he needed to get the cameras and video camera ready. I don't think he realized it was going to happen so fast. I started to get very cranky as the contractions intensified, and he continued to sleep. Some company would be nice. Contractions started coming closer together, 4-6 minutes apart, but some were coming right after another...and that worried me.

I got into the bath at about 2:15a.m. Contractions immediately slowed down, giving me a break and a chance to calm down. I had never been in a tub during any of my previous six births because I never was really drawn to it. (Although I always do spend a lot of time in the shower!), but holy cow the bath made contractions more bearable! Then the doula part of me started thinking that the contractions slowed down so much and I was worried that I got in the tub too early and now I wasn't in labor anymore. Oh geez! After one more strong contraction, I instantly realized that I was indeed still in labor.

I had to decide whether or not to call Dee. I still wasn't sure how long this was going to last, and I didn't want to call too soon (I hate calling people in the middle of the night!) and have her come over too early. But I decided to call her...I needed her there in case the babies (2 1/2 and 15 months) woke up because of my loud birthing noises. I got out of the bathtub and went straight into the shower in our master bedroom. I started feeling pressure, and I knew I had to go to the bathroom. Woo hoo! Baby was making its way down! So I took care of some bathroom business and then started to get really worried. The contractions were strong.

I had Charlie lay a huge bath towel on the floor between the shower and the toilet since I was going back and forth--I would stand in the shower between contractions and sit on the toilet during the contractions. It seemed that each time I stood up it would make another contraction start. This was all happening fast. I heard Dee arrive but I was having a contraction so we couldn't let her in. After it was done and Charlie let Dee in, I think the two of them got cameras and the video camera ready in the bedroom. I knew the baby was going to be born soon. I put the waterproof mat on the floor, in the same exact place where Caden was born 2 1/2 years earlier. That time the mat wasn't there. I asked Dee to turn off the lights and light the candles. Quickly, damn it!

I asked Charlie to feel for a head, to which he replied, "it feels like a shoulder." What? Don't say that! So I checked and it was just a squishy head. I asked (okay, demanded) a hot compress (disposable diaper filled with hot water)...quickly! To put on my perineum, a trick I learned with my first homebirth with a midwife. It feels so good and got me focused on what had to be done...push the baby out. I really disliked pushing in the past but this one was different, or else I have finally learned how to get it done. All I have to do is let go.

I asked Charlie if he wanted to see his baby. He said he was ready. I was standing holding myself up, one hand on the dresser, the other on the footboard and my feet completely off the floor and pushed the head out. Ah, relief! I leaned over Charlie's shoulder and he couldn't see the baby. He asked Dee to help hold me up, but I don't think there was enough room. Charlie was able to catch as I pushed the rest of the baby out and sat down on the floor. 3:33 AM.

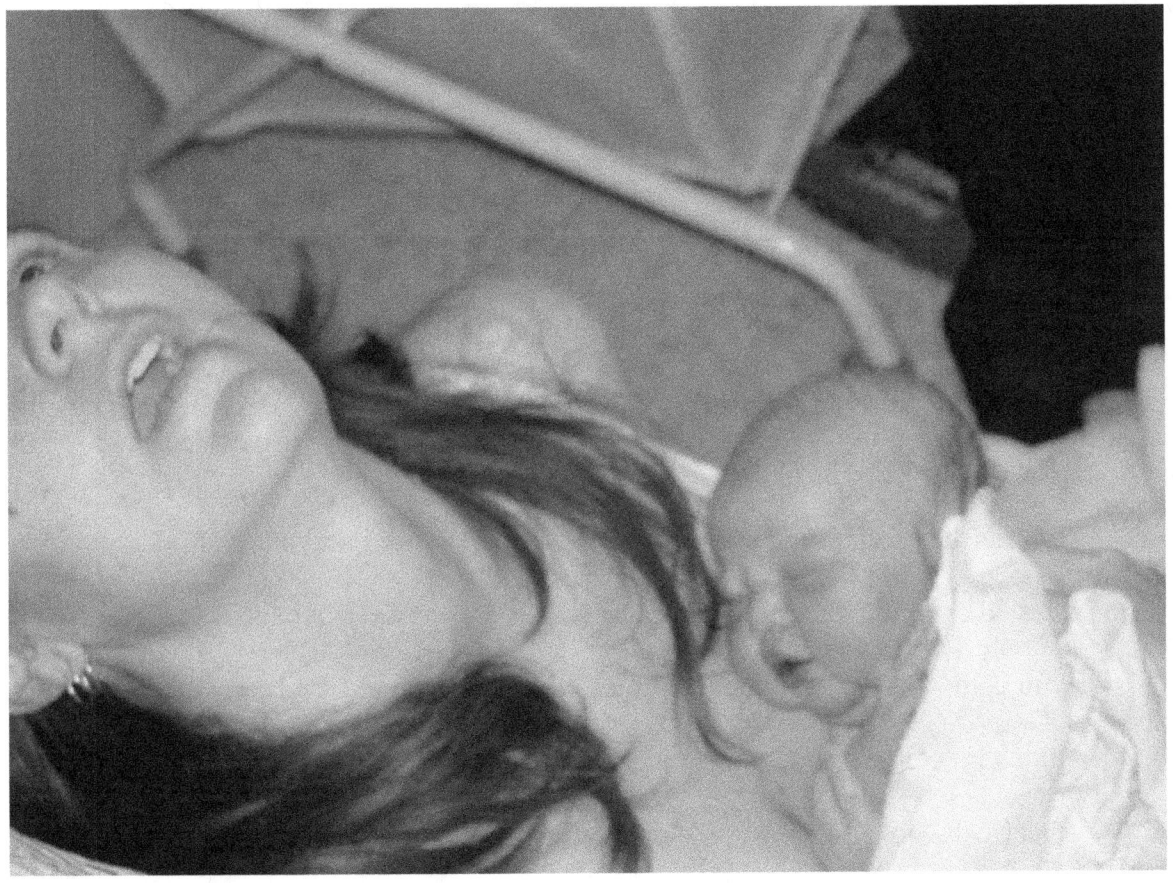

Woo hoo! It's over! That was a fast one! Then I realized I had to check to see if the baby was a boy or girl. I glanced and saw swollenness and thought to myself "How cool is that, my fifth boy!" I told Charlie "Look! Look!" and he replied, "You gave me my baby girl!" What? It's a girl? I asked Dee to turn on the light and checked again, and she really is a baby girl! Trust me; I have checked several times over the last few days...and she is still a girl!

I inspected her for a few minutes...she seemed smaller than my other babies. The placenta came within minutes, and that was smaller than my others, too. Charlie held her for a few minutes before we put her on the bed and clamped the cord. I cleaned up the towels and blankets and got into bed. I asked for breakfast and Dee thankfully ran to Denny's for me. I called work to let them know the news. We took some pictures and at about 5:30 a.m. I decided to get some sleep before the babies woke up.

Caden woke up first at about 7:00 a.m. He pranced into our bedroom and started climbing into our bed. Charlie said "Be careful -- we have a surprise for you up here." Caden found her laying between me and Charlie and said "Aw, I like her!" So sweet! Donovan woke up a little later and just wanted to poke her face. Silly boy! We went to church at 10:15 a.m., much to the surprise of most of the people attending that day. The baby received a special birthday blessing. We went out to lunch, and I stopped by my work to show her off. The older boys got home later and were surprised to finally have a sister!

It took us a few days to finally name her. We were trying to incorporate any form of "Elle" - for my middle name (Ellen,) Charlie's oldest sister's middle name (Ellen,) and Charlie's mother, Elsie. I don't know how we finally came up with it, but Ellyse came out of nowhere we had never considered it before, and Quinn for my fifth baby.

And finally, measurements were taken at the doctors the day after she was born. She was 7 lbs, 12 oz and 20 inches long. I think I got cheated out of the 8 oz of meconium she had already pooped out. I also checked in with my doctor the next day. He laughed at my request to do Charlie's vasectomy right there on the spot!

Mom	:Marlena
Dad	:Charlie
City/State	:Modesto, California
Age at birth	:31
Birth	:Seven
Baby's name	:Ellyse Quinn
Baby's Height	:20 inches
Baby's Weight	:7 lbs, 12 oz

Jordyn Rose

This was my third pregnancy, so you would think I would know what to expect. But somehow I still went through the last two weeks wondering if the prodromal labor I was having was ever going to progress into the "real" thing. My pregnancy was a healthy, fairly uneventful one. It was a real mix of my first two pregnancies. Around 18 weeks, I began having pubic pain and began to see a chiropractor every other week. This helped tremendously and I could actually stand on one leg, turn over in bed, get dressed, etc without screaming in pain that my pubic bone hurt.

Early in pregnancy I had read about the benefits of drinking red raspberry leaf tea, and how it tones the uterus and can help with a quick and easy labor, delivery and post partum period. I didn't order the herbs for the tea online until I was 30 weeks pregnant. I began drinking the tea at 31 weeks. I drank approximately one quart of the tea every day, religiously. I made it at night and drank it cold the next day. I like the taste, and figured it couldn't hurt to try. I was on a mission to see if it would really help shorten my labor. I had a 17-hour labor with Hayden and an 8-hour labor with Ellie so I wasn't a big believer that I could have a labor that was much shorter than that. I also began taking 2000mg of Evening Primrose Oil orally at 36 weeks to help soften my cervix.

At 37 weeks 3 days I began to feel my first set of prodromal labor and Braxton hick's contractions. The contractions began at 6:00 a.m. that morning and were happening every 10-30 minutes randomly throughout the day. By the next morning they were happening every ten minutes regularly. I had my husband and the kids go for a pretty long walk with me around the neighborhood and that seemed to help make them more regular. When we got home, I cleaned the house and waited for my midwives to arrive. They were already scheduled to come to the house that day for my prenatal appointment anyway. All throughout the day before and this day I had also been clearing out my bowels. I was convinced that this might actually be the beginning of labor for me, even though it was still early. Hayden was born ten days early, and Ellie was one week early so it wouldn't have been shocking for the baby to come this early. After my midwives arrived, these contractions petered out until later that evening. By the time I went to bed though, they were gone.

The next day I didn't have even one contraction, but the following day I felt very crampy all day and was having more contractions throughout the day. I went shopping with my mom and the kids at the outlets, hoping things would progress. Unfortunately I was just very uncomfortable all day and that night just before bed I began to feel better. This entire week my husband had been working 16-hour days trying to finish the job he was working on before baby's arrival. I think that mentally I did not want to have this baby while he was working so this may have inhibited things a bit too.

Throughout the next week, not much happened. The contractions I had been having went away completely. My best friend had her baby and I was so jealous. I continued drinking my tea every day, and taking the Evening Primrose Oil. I was also walking a couple miles every day and practically jumping my husband for some lovin' every night. By the time the baby was actually born, I think he was happy to hear he's getting a post partum break!

On Monday July 2nd, one day shy of 39 weeks, we went to see the midwives for my 39-week checkup. I asked to be checked and they said I was dilated to a very soft 4 cm! This was very encouraging, but I knew that it was possible to be 4 cm for days or even weeks and didn't want to get my hopes up too much that baby's arrival would be soon. Usually, the midwives bring the tub for the birth to the birth with them when they arrive. We had happened to bring the truck to that appointment and they offered for us to take a tub home with us if we wanted to. I jumped at the opportunity because I had already planned on waiting to the last minute to call them. But I was fearful that if I did I wouldn't be able to birth in the water, like I did with Ellie. This really put my mind at ease that I would be able to have water during labor, but not have to have the midwives there just waiting while I labored the entire time.

Tuesday, around mid afternoon I began having contractions that were more like cramps, very low in my pelvis. They were anywhere from 15-45 minutes apart and not very painful at all. We put the kids to bed that night and I decided to go for a quick walk around the block. My walk pretty much put a halt to my contractions, so I figured it would be at least another day before baby would arrive.

I called my mom that night about 10:30 p.m. to talk with her about how I was feeling about her being at the birth. She was at the birth of my first two, and this time around I was planning it to be just my husband, the kids and me. Which she already knew this, but had been making comments about how she was hurt by this. I wanted to labor alone and not have the pressure of someone waiting for the baby to arrive and the baby not arriving quick enough for everyone else. I think she had been feeling a bit hurt that I did not want her there, and I just wanted to explain that it wasn't that I didn't want her there, but that I didn't want anyone there. I didn't want to share this birth like I had the other two, and wanted it to be my own. I think we finally came to an understanding where she wasn't feeling hurt anymore and I didn't have to feel guilty about not wanting her to be there.

A little bit after my phone call with my mom I requested my husband come to the bedroom for some lovin'. I was a woman obsessed with doing everything I could to encourage this baby to join us! Not five minutes after we were done I felt a very intense contraction down very low in my pelvis that radiated around into my lower back/upper bottom area. This was strange for me because with my other two labors my contractions were felt higher up and took over my whole belly. These weren't in my "belly" at all, just down super low. Exactly two minutes later I felt another one and I had to yell for my husband to come back into the bedroom. For the next ten minutes or so they were coming strong every two minutes. I was moaning through them and I had to have Obee pushing hard, applying pressure on my lower back, just above my bottom throughout each one. I'm not sure how long they were lasting...maybe 45 seconds each. Obee was practically begging me to call my mom to come over. We had a little discussion about it and he said that he needed her here. He was a little scared I think, and unlike myself, he realized that things were going to happen quickly and my mom lives closer to us than the midwives do. The contractions were coming so quickly together, that I honestly wanted my mom there at that moment as well. I should have known I would want my mom there!

After hanging up with her, Obee insisted we call the midwives, but I was still a bit reluctant to call them. It was 11:45 p.m. by this time, and I thought that maybe this was just another set of contractions that would peter out. Luckily I agreed to call them. When I called, they had only been asleep an hour, because they had just returned home from two other births in the last 24 hours. They asked if my water had broken and asked if I could check myself to see if I was dilated anymore. I told them it hadn't broken and that I was fine, but to hold on a second. I threw Obee the phone as another contraction came over me. Obee told me that as soon as they heard me moaning they said, "We'll be right there." and hung up the phone.

After hanging up the phone with the midwives, everything happened so quickly that it is very fuzzy in my mind. It was all so surreal, and I felt almost like I was watching it from the outside. Obee began getting the tub set up and I hopped in the shower. I wanted to be clean before labor and have my hair done up in a nice bun so that it wouldn't get all frizzy after laboring many hours in the tub. Now I think back to what a waste of time that was. Taking a shower was precious time that water could have been filling up the birthing tub! The hose to fill the tub hooks up through the shower. Washing my hair through contractions wasn't the funniest thing either. I really wanted to be on my hands and knees or bent over on the bed, but there wasn't enough room for any of that in the shower.

I honestly don't remember getting dressed and doing my hair after the shower, but I did have a shirt on so I must have done it at some point. At this point in my labor, I only had about thirty seconds between contractions. They were coming one after another. I remember actually saying out loud, "I can do this...I can do this...I can do this." I had to remind myself that I could.

I knew the baby was very low at this point and really began to think that it was going to arrive before my mom and the midwives. I began to have a bloody show and luckily had already placed a towel under me. I was on my hands and knees moaning and my poor husband was running around like a chicken with his head cut off trying to do everything himself. He was hooking up the tub, getting me water, checking on the kids, and still having to be back every thirty seconds to push on my back! He was amazing!

Somewhere between all of this my mom and the midwives arrived. About five minutes after they all arrived, they said that I could finally get into the tub. It wasn't even half full yet, but it was enough to help tremendously. I thought I wasn't going to be able to get in though, because I felt like my body wouldn't move from the spot on the floor where I already was. The water was amazing! It helped through those last contractions so much and I was at ease knowing I had made it to the tub in time. As soon as I got into the tub I was feeling pushy and knew the baby was coming quickly. Luckily my mom knew to go get the kids out of bed, as they really didn't want to miss the birth and I wanted them to see it as well. My body felt an overwhelming urge to push and I reached down to see if I could feel the baby there after I pushed. I could definitely feel something, but it wasn't just the baby. It was the baby in her water sack still intact. It felt like a big squishy balloon. With the next contraction, my mom came back in the room with the kids and I pushed as hard as I could. I reached down to be able to catch her as she emerged. I had a million different thoughts during this last push; it's just amazing to me how many different things I was thinking of in such a quick period of time. I felt her head come out and decided to just continue pushing the rest of her out in one big push. I didn't want to frighten my other kids with another big yell like I was making with this push. I had prepared them before the birth that mommy would yell, but that I would be okay, etc. The big moan that I let out with that last push surprised even me though. It felt better to make the noises though. As my baby's feet emerged, her water bag broke and I lifted her up to me.

I could hear Hayden asking if it was a boy or girl and I wanted to know first, so I reached down real quick and felt that she was a girl! Everyone was so surprised because daddy had been so sure that it was a boy and he had convinced everyone else of that too. He even almost had me convinced, but I kept going back to the dream I had in pregnancy of birthing a baby girl. It really showed me that I should trust my instincts more and that intuitively I did know it was a girl!

Jordyn Rose was born at 12:45 a.m. on July 4th; just one hour and fifteen minutes after my labor began. She weighed 7 lbs 8 oz and was 20.5 inches long. Less than two minutes after coming out, Jordyn was smacking her lips ready to nurse. She nursed for a good twenty minutes in the tub. We stayed in the tub this whole time, and then birthed the placenta before getting out. She is such a sweet little pumpkin and so very loved by her big brother and sister too.

Dad	: Obee
Birth	: Third
Baby's name	: Jordyn Rose
Baby's Height	: 20.5 inches
Baby's Weight	: 7lbs 8oz

Soterius

My birth story is wonderful. My husband and I caught the baby at our home in the bathtub. My baby was born three weeks early and our birthing pool was due to arrive any day...but Soterius didn't want to wait that long to come. I began to go into labor at around 11:00 p.m. at night. My contractions weren't severe, and they felt like painful gas at the worst. I didn't have any pain medications and I didn't feel the need to cry out at all. At around five in the morning I felt the contractions coming closer and closer together. My husband then implemented the acupressure points we had researched to help the baby drop and out he came. He was born in the water and didn't even start to cry until a few minutes after. Because I was in the bathtub the whole time my pain was minimal and I also didn't have any tearing. I was able to ride my bike two weeks later. It was the most amazing and beautiful thing I have ever been a part of.

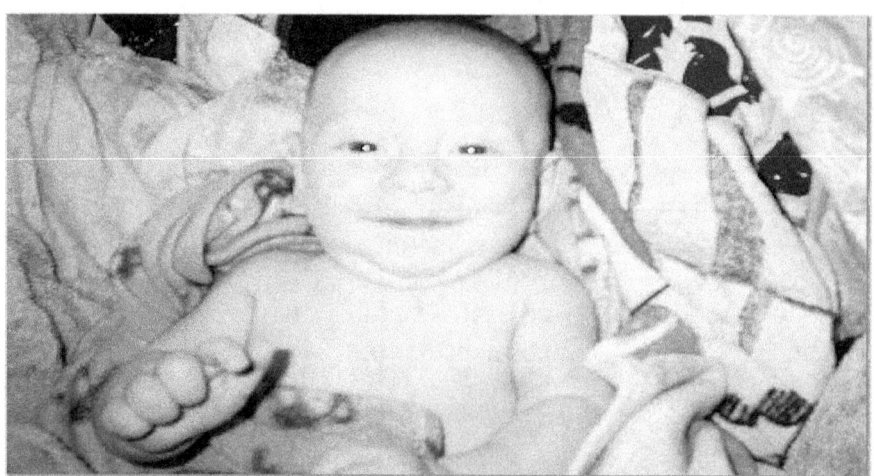

Linkin Alexander

I had my regular weekly appointment with the midwife at about 5:00 p.m. and everything was great. She said the baby had dropped and my blood pressure and urine were good too. She had wanted to do the Strep B test and since she would be in the area I asked her to check me. I had been having bad backaches that I could time for about a week. Well it turns out I was 90% effaced and 2 cm dilated. She said the baby was plastered on my cervix and wasn't budging. We all joked that the baby might come earlier than expected and made a guess of Sept.13th.

I went home and at about 8:00 p.m. I noticed that I was having regular contractions every ten minutes or so. They were noticeable but I could still talk through them. I didn't tell my husband because I figured it was a false alarm. At 9:00 p.m. my water broke! It had meconium in it so I called the midwife right away. She said as long as it doesn't look like pea soup and the texture is very watery then we are fine. It was like water so all was good. She said to get some rest and call when the contractions are five minutes apart lasting one min. She told me to get some rest to save my energy for the big day.

Well my husband and I were totally unprepared and didn't even have a stopwatch. I knew the contractions were coming pretty steady though. I don't know why we don't have any darn clocks in the house. We needed a hose for the birth tub too so we decided to go to Wal-Mart before heading to bed. On the way to Wal-Mart I was having contractions every 3-5 min lasting 50 seconds. I could still talk through them and just kept thinking oh man this is going to be so hard if it starts out this intense. I called my midwife and she just told me to relax and that labor can start out a little intense but die down quickly.

We got what we needed and headed home. I lost all sense of time right about now. I wanted to get in the shower and that lasted maybe ten minutes. My husband kept saying, "Let's just lay down and try to sleep". I was so angry because there was no way I was sleeping. The contractions were strong and about two minutes apart by now.

I think around 10:30 p.m. I needed to sit on the toilet backwards. My husband told me I was having contractions every two minutes and they were lasting 90 seconds. I was in denial big time and I think at this point my saying was "This is going fast. This is not normal. This is going fast". I said "Call the midwife right now". I was vocalizing through the contractions so loud and couldn't hold back. The weird thing was I didn't think I was in labor. It only hurt way down low and I was always told that it would start at the top of your uterus and contract down. My husband kept saying, "I think you're in transition" and I was laughing at him because I didn't even think I was in labor. So my husband called the midwife and told her she needs to come right away. I remember at this point thinking that she would come over and I would only be 3 cm dilated. I thought to myself "Ok if this is what labor is like I can't do this...props to all the natural birthers out there but oh my goodness this is hard".

Next thing I know I feel the contractions doubling. There is no break and the energy was just so strong. I started crying and told my husband that I wasn't getting a break. I was way gone in labor land. My body was pushing. I couldn't control it but I didn't tell my husband because the midwife wasn't there.

My husband said that I should go on the exercise ball because it will calm me down. I tried it for maybe three seconds and then hopped on the bed on all fours. I just did what my body was telling me to do. I lifted my bum up high and pushed my face into the mattress. At this point I was clearly pushing and the midwife just arrived. She walked in and said, "Wow this is serious!" I was naked and didn't care. She told me she could hear my pushes and they were just what I needed to do. She finally got all set up and just told me to listen to my body. I did and my body pushed so hard. I had no control and felt very animal like. I was growling so loud I shocked myself. Even at this point I was saying, "This is fast, I don't think I can do it". The midwife said "You are going to have your baby out in ten minutes so just push". The ring of fire was intense as most people say. I remember asking every five seconds...."Is he out yet? How much longer? Is he out yet?" Then finally the midwife said, "Yes he's out!"

I flipped over and the midwife put him on my chest. He was crying and just so gorgeous. I got all cleaned up.... hopped in the shower then tried breastfeeding which is going great. Oh and I didn't have any tears at all. We are so in love with him and he's just perfect.

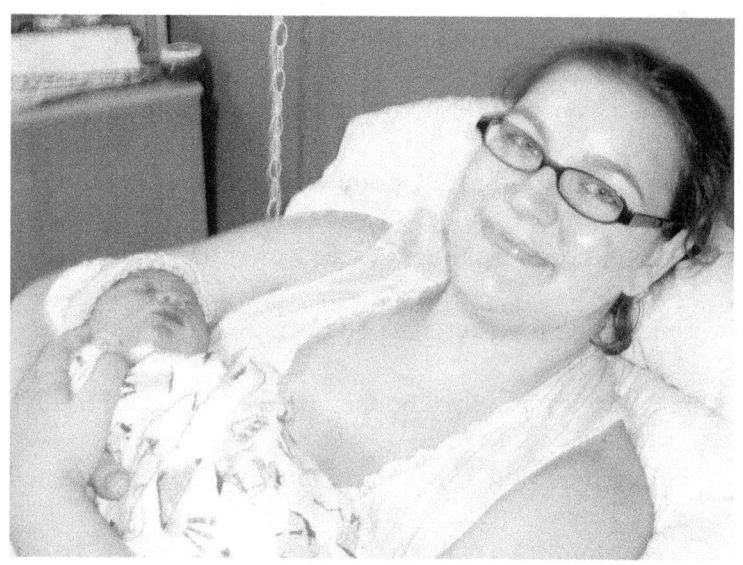

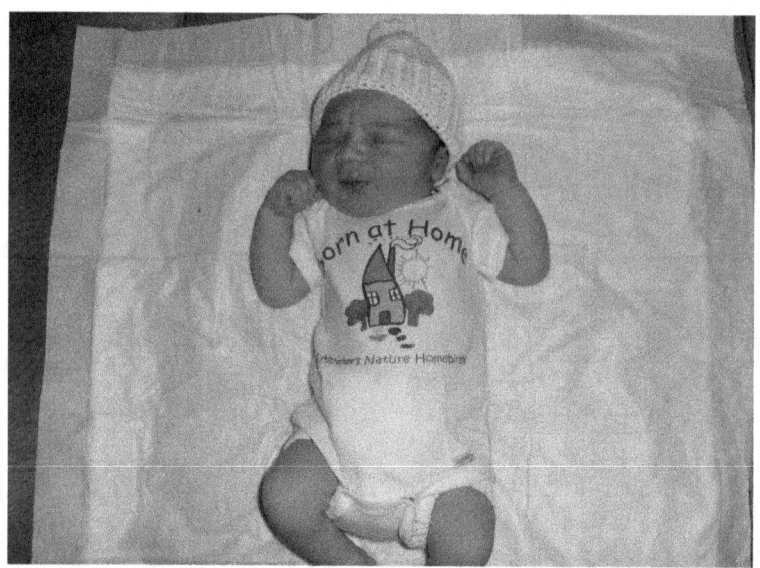

Mom	: Terri
Dad	: David
City State	: Florida
Age at birth	: 25
Birth	: First
Baby's name	: Linkin Alexander
Baby's Height	: 20'
Baby's Weight	: 8lb 0 oz

Maeve

It's seven thirty in the morning and here I am up and ready to go. It's funny, my husband Michael's sister Jane had this big monologue around Christmas time about how you don't just have a baby and *become* a mother. What she was trying to say was more along the lines of mothers keeping an identity after the birth of a 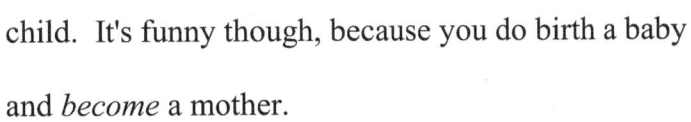 child. It's funny though, because you do birth a baby and *become* a mother.

For example, I loved to sleep. Note the past tense. Then I had Maeve, I didn't sleep for six weeks and I didn't miss it. My body did, but I wouldn't have had it any other way. Now that she's eight weeks, she sleeps from 10:00 p.m. to 8.30 or 9:00 in the morning, waking up a few times to eat and be changed, but never really "waking" up. It's funny to be on the other end of the mother-child relationship. As a kid you wonder, "How can mom be up so early?" but as a mom, once you've gotten eight hours, you're ready to go- even if it is seven thirty.

Michael is going to St. John's College in Santa Fe, NM. We leave at the beginning of August. I'm excited to be in a larger pool of people (though the school is really small, only 700 students). Santa Fe is the third largest art hub in the country, though it's a relatively small city. I don't know that much about it and it's pretty much a leap of faith, but I think it'll work out.

About my birth, I'll try and sketch out some here, it's hard to format all the memories I have into a linear story. It's like trying to write down a dream. I was in labor for three days or so before Maeve was born. This sounds bad, but in truth, I was up and about and walking around for almost all of it. The only thing was I didn't *realize* I was in labor. It sounds funny, but I had gotten so used to new physical sensations and discomforts during pregnancy that not being able to get comfortable anywhere, and having my "practice" contractions pick up didn't send off any bells in my head.

After two days of this increasing energy (I got really spacey) I realized that this was it. Mike and I spent the day in the house playing board games and watching movies. Toward the end of the day my mother called and offered to come over with some food. Now, I had had many birth plans at this point. The basics were always the same, homebirth, tub there for the option of water birth, or just help with the contractions, lots of moving around and taking different positions. The thing that had changed was who was supposed to be there. In essence, it's impossible to understand labor without having done it.

At first only Michael and I and the midwife were going to be there. Then the midwife wanted to bring her assistant. Then they suggested that I have someone there to make soup of; to run around and do whatever else needed to be done. We couldn't think of anyone, so decided against it. Well, then one of the midwives actually realized what a homebirth on Lopez in December meant; possible very bad weather. She had a pretty thorough freak out about emergencies and transportation, etc. Unfortunately at this point I was past six months so it was too late to find a new midwife, especially one who would come to Lopez. We contacted a woman we knew and asked her if she would be an emergency person, in case the midwives couldn't make it to the island. She said yes, but then decided she wanted to be there *instead* of the midwives. She did her best to convince me not to call them, and she began to show up at our house unannounced whenever she felt like it. This whole time my mother kept asking to be there, and I kept telling her no.

When the time came to figure out what to do, I called the midwives. The hesitancy there was not wanting someone to come who was freaked out about our situation, we decided that if she was terrible we would tell her to leave, or go to a hospital. My mother, who was there just to say hi and drop off soup, ended up staying because I didn't want her to leave. My sister April was even there, because at the last minute it sounded good.

The midwife came on the last ferry and arrived at the house (Michael's uncle's cabin) at about midnight. I was just then at the point of not being able to pay attention to a game of backgammon, abandoning my second game in a row. I was really worried that Ali the midwife would show up and I wouldn't be dilated at all. Then everyone would be disappointed and I would feel foolish. I hoped I would be at least three centimeters. As soon as she got situated Ali checked me and I was *seven* centimeters.

From then on out things are an increasing blur. I walked around the house in circles, bounced on a big exercise ball and laid down for a few naps. (I didn't actually sleep). I hit transition at about ten centimeters. I was in transition for a really long time, which was interesting. I think that this was the time when I had to get some emotional things out of the way before I could have the baby. In hindsight I realize that what I had to let go of was *being* the baby. I had to let myself whine and complain and be bossy until I got it all out. This was hard on everyone else, because they didn't really understand what I was going through (Except for my Mom). They were really compassionate, but worried that I was "losing" it. I wasn't in the space to explain anything to them, so I just left everyone else to their own devices.

Her assistant was amazing. She did almost everything so I suppose she was the real midwife. She was kind and patient and she monitored the baby a lot, which was important to us. At the end of transition Ali gave me some homeopathies, to "speed things up". After that I got in the tub. The water was wonderful; it took all the weight and made me float. I could easily change position, and my backache was no longer crippling. Up until this point, Mike, My mom and April had been taking turns rubbing my lower back hard. The sensations in my womb weren't painful, just like menstrual cramps, but the backache was a killer. After a few moments (in my time, not earth time, so it was probably an hour) the contractions mellowed out and started to transition into the urge to push. This is what transition means, and it can last for anywhere from a minute to four hours, like mine did.

Then I got to push. This was the fun part because now I was doing something. I pushed for about four hours. It's interesting work because you have to learn how to push, and also because I could feel the baby come down a little, then slip back a little. It's very two steps forward one step back. When Maeve came down the birth canal enough I could feel her head, very soft. At the last few pushes Michael hopped in the tub with me, and out she came. Her feet were stuck, so Mike had to give a little pull. He liked that part. She lay on my chest with her eyes scrunched tightly closed, breathing well but not crying. I held her away from me for a moment and she gave a nice couple of hollers. When I put her back on me she quieted down at once.

It's funny, for about ten hours I had my eyes shut tightly because everything was very out of focus, and I could hardly hear a word anyone said. But as soon as Maeve was settled on me, I looked up to see everything sharply in focus and said " Now who's gonna make me a sandwich?" After that I handed the baby to Mike (who was out of the tub at this point) and I got out and lay down in the bed. After everyone left I took a shower and we all went to bed. We slept well, because birth was really hard work for everyone.

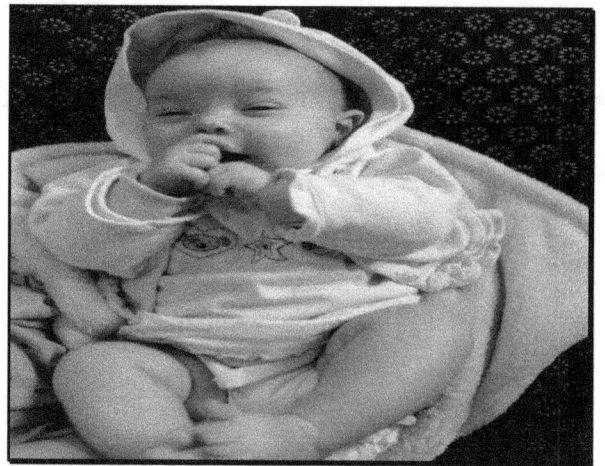

Mommy	:Crystal
Daddy	:Micheal
City State	:Lopez Island, WA
Age at birth	:21
Birth	:1
Baby's Name	:Mauve
Baby's Height	:19.5 inches
Baby's Weight	:7lbs 12oz

Sophia's Wisdom

The story of Sophia's birth has to start with Simon, whose planned natural hospital birth center birth turned into a planned cesarean in labor because he was persistently breech. I was terribly disappointed by the loss of the natural and gentle birth I had wanted for him, and traumatized by an awful, inadequately anesthetized surgical delivery and utterly insulting "care" in the hospital. I spent the next year reading, learning, sleeping and breathing birth and VBAC, and knew with certainty from before I conceived that my next baby would be born at home. Lily's pregnancy was peaceful; I had great midwives, enjoyed preparing for birth with Hypnobabies, and looked forward with complete confidence to my expected HBAC. But when my water broke in early labor, it was nothing but gushing blood and clots, and we ended up with an ambulance transport and emergency cesarean under general anesthetic. I was deeply grateful that Lily was healthy despite a major placental abruption, but devastated at the loss of everything I had hoped for her and for myself in her birth – it killed me that I wasn't even consciously there when she came into the world.

When I became pregnant around a year later, it was a bit of a surprise. This time around I had no confident plans, no sure hopes. I felt that my intuition had been broken and scarred by Lily's birth, and I was filled with fear. My husband was uncomfortable with considering any out-of-hospital options; my mother had begged me not to try again at home. Despite my fear I knew I couldn't plan an elective repeat cesarean; it just wasn't in me to do it. So I went back to the OB whom I had seen as backup during Lily's pregnancy, and just planned to try for a vba2c in the hospital…with my intuition and faith shaken, it seemed easiest to just go with what other people thought was best. But as time went on, and I tried to visualize myself going to the hospital to birth, it just didn't feel right. There was no one who believed in me there, I would be only a big medical-legal risk walking through the halls, trying to fight the system and birth my baby at the same time. I found new research showing that rates of complication after two cesareans were not significantly different than the risks after one…. and more that showed the climbing risks to my health and life with each subsequent cesarean…and found that there was a hospital within two miles of my new home in case of emergency. And I knew that if no one else believed in me, my midwives would. So as hard as it was to get over the fear of doing things the same way as I had when they had ended so traumatically, everything was pointing me toward giving homebirth another go. At 24 weeks I called the midwives and made an appointment, and we started on the path toward what would be Sophia's birth.

Around 30 weeks I began to suspect that I was carrying another breech baby – felt that hard, telltale noggin right up under my ribs. At my 32-week prenatal, Bridget confirmed that she thought babe was breech too. We talked briefly about her comfort with breech births, and she talked about their hands-off approach and the more than a dozen breech homebirths they had attended in the last few years. I wasn't sure what I would decide yet if the baby stayed breech. I made a chiropractic appointment that same day, started doing tilting exercises, and started reading the book "Breech Birth" that Bridget had lent me. After reviewing the research, thinking and praying, and seeing that even ACOG had changed their guidelines in favor of breech birth since Simon was born, I decided to continue with the homebirth plan, though not without trepidation.

I had an ultrasound at 36 weeks to confirm that the butt and not the feet were presenting, and that the baby's head was flexed, and all looked favorable for a vaginal breech. I was still seeing the OB as shadow care, to maintain relationships in case of transfer, and I decided to allow him to try a version at 37 weeks. I declined an epidural so that I could maintain sensation and tell him to stop if it felt wrong. He got baby's head about halfway down, but she was bracing with her feet, and on the second attempt it did feel wrong and I stopped the process. She quickly made her way back to her favorite comfy position, breech and left sacrum anterior. I did not choose to share our homebirth plan outside of my immediate family – really just my husband – so the OB assumed we would have a cesarean, though I did not agree to schedule one at that time.

I really thought that the baby would come early, maybe around 38 weeks, as I had heard that breech babies often do. And I hoped she would, because I was concerned about having another big babe (Simon and Lily had both been 9+

pounds). But I was carrying small and Wendy said she felt that baby was probably around 6 pounds in the 37th week, and she didn't seem to be going anywhere. By 40 weeks I was antsy, having bouts of prodromal contractions off and on for several weeks, but she still felt to be around 7.5 lbs, still within reasonable guidelines for a breech birth, so we hung in there. I saw the shadow OB at 40 weeks 2 days, and got the hard sell for a scheduled cesarean a.s.a.p. I refused, but the doctor called on Thursday, March 29, saying my cesarean was scheduled for Friday the 30th. I had my husband call her back and tell her we wouldn't be coming.

When I woke from a nap that afternoon, I found an incredibly long message from her on the answering machine, the upshot of which was that her schedule and 'the best interest of me and my baby' required that I be there in the morning for the cesarean, which was still on the books. I found this incredibly stressful and called my husband to decide what to do about it…and while I was talking to him around 3:00 p.m. I found I was having contractions that were stopping me in my tracks, every few minutes. By the end of the conversation I asked him to come home because I was having trouble paying attention to the kids and dealing with the contractions at the same time. I wasn't sure that it was really labor, since I had had a few bouts of pretty tough contractions that hadn't gone anywhere over the past few weeks, but I definitely needed his help.

Eric got home around 4:00 p.m., and I called Wendy to tell her what was going on. She suggested I take an extra dose of calcium/magnesium and extra water, because that would calm things down if it were just an irritated uterus but wouldn't stop the real thing. My mother-in-law came around 6:00 p.m. to take Simon and Lily to her house, and I spent the evening just sort of puttering around between contractions, watched a movie with Eric, and had some dinner. We started noticing the contractions coming closer together and stronger, and there was bloody show along with them, so I called Wendy again around 8:00 p.m. and she said it sounded like it was time to have a baby. Eric decided to go get some rest, and I lay on the couch listening to hypnosis scripts and breathing through the contractions until Wendy came around 11:00 p.m. I found that the Hypnobabies plan of being "Loose and limp and relaxed" during the "Wonderful birthing waves" just wasn't doing it for me – I could not remain still at all, had to rock, bounce, sway through them. Things continued like this for several more hours…since Bridget was out of town Maryanne, a midwife from Michigan, was coming down, and she arrived at some point…lots of tough contractions 2 or 3 minutes apart, and I decided to get in the tub around 1:00 a.m. or 2:00 a.m.. At this point it really seemed like things might go pretty quickly, but it wasn't to be. I was in there for a while until I started dozing off between contractions, got up to go to the bathroom, came back and sat in a recliner and things started to space out a lot. I was still dozing in between contractions, and Wendy suggested that I go down and get in bed while things were slacked off so that I could get some rest.

So I went down to bed and actually got decent rest between contractions, as they had spaced out to maybe every 10-15 minutes. Wendy came in every hour or so to listen to the babe, who was doing fine, and around 7:00 a.m. on Friday I got up and Wendy said they had another mom in labor. She asked if I was willing to be checked to see where things stood so they could decide where to go and when, and I was fine with that as I really wanted to know whether all the contractions were doing anything or not. She found that I was fully effaced and 5-6 cm, but that my cervix was still really posterior with the butt not applied very well, which explained the slow progress. She pulled the cervix forward and suggested I stay upright as much as possible – and also strongly suggested that I eat a decent breakfast, as it could really take a while longer. Eric went out for eggs and breakfast stuff, and I ate as much as I could though nothing was really appetizing. Contractions were still strong but far apart, 10-15 minutes. It was a beautiful morning and Maryanne suggested we take a walk to see if that would move things along. They did pick up while I was walking, but not by much. The midwives decided to leave to check on the other mom, and left us with the Doppler to keep checking baby. I was fine with this as I was starting to feel like a watched pot that was never going to boil.

Eric and I spent the next few hours just hanging out, watched a weird German movie about a girl who believed she was possessed by the devil, and took another walk. Wendy and Maryanne came back around 4:00 p.m. to check on us – the other mom hadn't yet had her baby yet either. I got checked and things were still pretty much the same, again with the posterior cervix. They left again to give us privacy. We went out to Blockbuster and rented yet more movies (and I had to hide behind the shelves and bend over rocking with my hands on knees to get through the contractions in between searching for a good flick), and picked up some Chinese food for dinner. My dad came to pick up our laundry, and I was a little nervous because we hadn't shared the plan with him or my mother, but I was fine during the brief time he was at the house – I really wanted my labor to be private until the baby was here.

I was getting discouraged and worried...even though Wendy had assured me that the baby was fine, and that as long as vitals were good and I could eat drink and pee, we could stick with it for as long as it took. Before she left she had told me the story of another VBAC mom who had labored 3 days, 3 centimeters a day, only between 7:00 p.m. and 3:00 a.m., and the baby was born at 3:00 a.m. on the third day. I held on to that story, and to the 80+ hours VBAC that I remembered reading of – but I also had doubts that this was really ever going to go anywhere or would ever pick up again. I had shared with Maryanne my remembering the Dr. Michel Odent saying that breech births should be smooth and progressive or you should give it up, and I wasn't sure that was happening. She told me too that baby was fine, and that 6 cm was definitely progress, that this was my third baby but my first vaginal birth and there was nothing too unusual about what was going on.

I was also really starting to miss Simon and Lily, and just felt bored and discouraged and tired. I talked to Eric about how I was feeling, that I was worried, wondered whether I should just give it up and go have that cesarean after all, that I didn't know what was going on. He just listened, asked why I was feeling that way and whether I thought there was real reason for concern. I decided that I would hang out a few more hours and try to figure out what was going on. I called Wendy around 11:00 p.m. still feeling pretty distraught, feeling like this had been going on forever with no change in sight, and once again she reassured me that everything was going fine except for a poky labor, and said she would come again to check on us when they finished with the other mom's birth ("She lapped you" Eric said…oh well), in a few hours.

I cried to Eric again about missing the kids, about feeling discouraged, about not knowing what to do and that I just wanted them home. The labor was manageable; I could do it for days if it kept going that way. But I couldn't stand missing them and putting everyone's lives on hold for so long. So despite its being almost midnight, we decided we would just go get the kids. Eric told his mom, who had assumed we were going to the hospital, about our homebirth plan. He told her that it was just going slower than expected, and we didn't know how long it would take and we wanted the kids at home. She was very understanding and okay about it. We picked up the sleeping kiddos and put them in the car, and labor started to pick up again on the drive home. We put Simon and Lily in bed, and Eric went to lie down. I stayed in the living room trying to rest on the couch, with contractions coming every 5 or 6 minutes again. I was encouraged that maybe things would finally get moving. When Maryanne and Wendy arrived, I asked that they check me again, and Wendy found I was at around 7.5 cm, cervix still posterior. I was definitely heartened that there was some progress, however slow. They decided to stay and sleep and see where things were in the morning. The rest of the night is kind of a blur, just moving around the house to deal with the contractions…I lay down for a while, paced for a while, rocked on the ball, sat on the toilet, lay down again. Most of my active laboring time I was alone, with everyone sleeping, and that was okay.

The kids started waking up around 7:00 a.m. (we're all the way to Saturday morning now). Lily got to nurse on the couch for a while as much as I could stand it. Wendy suggested we call Mary to come watch them since I was continuing to labor pretty heavily. I retreated into our bedroom while Eric went out and took care of the kids. I just kept it up, leaning over the bed, trying to lie on my side since I was so tired (didn't work), more bouncing, and more rocking. At some point in the morning I got checked again and Wendy said I was at nine or so, but with an anterior lip, since the cervix still didn't want to stay up front. She told me how to hold it myself, and I tried to do that as much as I could during some contractions and in between. Contractions were coming faster and harder and less of a break and it had just been going on so long and I still didn't believe it would ever really go anywhere or that I would really get a baby, and I started getting really weepy, sobbing that I couldn't do this shit anymore…which of course I was assured was 'just transition'. I decided to go up and get in the tub again, stayed there who knows how long…by around noon I had made it to 10 cm. Maryanne said "You did it, you're there…" but still I didn't believe it. Things slowed down some then, I was just waiting on an urge to push but remembered that there was sometimes a "Rest and be thankful" stage between dilating and pushing, and I was all in favor of that since I was exhausted. I just relaxed and dozed between contractions, which spaced out some…drank a smoothie that Wendy made, got out of the tub and sat looking out a window in a squeaky desk chair that was just right for rocking during contractions. Started feeling like the babe was moving lower, like I could feel her ratcheting downward millimeter by millimeter during contractions. But it was still kind of chilled out just then.

Then I became aware of a commotion outside the room. I was confused to hear the voice of my mother, who was definitely not invited. She had a vicious and rageful tone in her voice, and was threatening that "They have five minutes to clear out of here or I am calling the police…I knew you would do this…I love my daughter enough to stop her from killing herself'. It was insane and I couldn't believe it was truly happening. In a fog I tried to take the phone away from her, but Eric said no and that he would handle it, and told her to leave the house. He called the police because she would not leave. She called the paramedics. I stayed upstairs in a strange state of calm. Decided I had better put on some clothes, so I got on a matching pair of clean pajamas and got my glasses. Mary came up to check on me, and assured me that Simon and Lily were okay and that Melissa and Wendy had left per Eric's request. I heard the fire trucks and ambulance pull up outside, and I wondered whether there would soon be people rushing into the house, but nothing happened. I pictured different scenes of what could happen next, but I knew that we had a right to refuse treatment and that Eric would stand up for us. Labor pretty much stopped at this point, thank God – the fight-or-flight response kicked in just when it was needed. I went downstairs and nursed Lily for a few minutes.

Wendy called and told Mary to tell Eric to request a waiver that we could sign to send away unwanted emergency personnel, and a few minutes later he brought in the papers saying I needed to sign them in front of the paramedics and they would leave. So I marched outside in my nice pajamas with Lily on my hip and looked at about fifteen paramedics, firefighters, a couple of police officers, and my mother, all standing outside our front gate. I said to them that I did not require their services and that I had not called for them, that I wanted them to leave and would be happy to sign whatever they needed to make that happen. One of them, an officious lady EMT, began a speech about killing my baby, plenty of shroud-waving indeed, and that she needed to take my blood pressure. I said "No, I don't consent to any treatment at this time, I will go to the hospital myself if I feel it is needed, like any other pregnant woman in the world" EMT said she had to call a doctor because of the "apparent life-threatening condition" that we were in…I asked "what's life-threatening here, I'm fine" and she blustered something about breech blah blah. She got an OB from the hospital on the phone and held it out to me asking would I please speak with her; I said that I would call my doctor when I chose to do so and no thank you. I just didn't want to give them any in that I had consented to *anything at all*. So the EMT said I just had to "Sign here so that if you and your baby die I won't lose my job." I said, "Sure, we wouldn't want that", signed on the dotted line that I refused services, and went back inside. Incredibly, as I turned to go in, my mother called out "Cassidy, you owe me the courtesy of at least coming to talk to me." I replied that she had owed me the courtesy of not invading my privacy and my home and threatening my family, and I didn't feel I owed her anything. Within ten minutes or so they pulled out…it took the police a few minutes longer, and my mother continued to sit on the curb in front of my home. Mary told me how she had shoved her way into the house, and she had threatened me that if the midwives came back she would call the police again. Since we live in a state where CPMs are not licensed, we were concerned that their presence would give cause for police to come in, so we decided that it would be safer to go somewhere else to have the baby. Mary said we were welcome to come to their house. So we prepared to "transport" for our homebirth at someone else's house.

My mother was still parked outside our house, and after her wild behavior and threats, we felt there was every chance that she would try to follow us and call the police again. We got all the birth supplies that we could gather out to the car – the midwives had left everything and gone home to switch cars in case their license plates had been noted, and would meet us at Mary's. As we all walked out to get into the car, my mother started her car, and I realized that if she started out then, she could get around behind our garage before we could get the kids in and get out. So I decided to go speak with her while Eric got everyone situated and pulled the car out and ready to take off. I expressed to her how sorry I was that she had done this, and that it was going to burn bridges in our family that I didn't know that I would be able to repair even if I wanted to. She said that if the baby or I died, she would never forgive herself if she hadn't done something to stop it. I said she had no reason to believe that we were going to die, that life has risks, that I have made my choices based on plenty of thought and care, but that this was not the time or place to discuss them. And then I made a run for the car. We went around a bit of a long way, stopped in a secluded parking lot for a bit to make sure she wasn't following, and then went on to Mary's. Later I told Eric that it was as though all of my own fears and doubts literally showed up on my doorstep in extreme physical form, with flashing lights and death threats, and I got to physically face them down and affirm that I was going to do this – and once this was done, the final chapter of this birth saga could begin.

And of course, labor picked up again in the car on the way there. We checked baby with the Doppler as soon as we arrived and she was still ticking along, despite all the stress and excitement we were feeling. We got there about 5:00 p.m., and Mary's husband had set up their bedroom for us, covered the bed and chairs, lots of towels ready. Simon and Lily went to play in the playroom, and Mary and her family and Maryanne and Wendy arrived a few minutes later. They came and hugged us, talked about what a time we had had and how sorry they were, and then Wendy told me that it was pretty likely that my cervix had closed up some. Mary had sent in some arnica 200c that I should take every 15 minutes for the next hour to deal with any cervical swelling, and we would see where things were in an hour or so. So just back to laboring, I wandered around the bedroom, got in and out of the shower, walked around the backyard stopping to rock and moan. Around 6:30 a.m. Maryanne checked on the baby and me; we were at 7-8 centimeters. Wendy told me "You are doing this, you are giving your baby a gentle birth just like you dreamed, you're okay and we are here for you." And I was back to transition for the second go-round. More crying, and this time it wasn't only that I couldn't do it and it hurt too much but that it was absolutely not fair that I had to do this part again! I had been doing this for days! I remember thinking that I would totally transfer and have a cesarean just for the pain relief, if only it wouldn't take such a long time riding in the car to get there. I just felt frantic with the pain though, there was less and less of a break in between and I couldn't find anything that made it better…no matter what position I was in I felt trapped when a contractions would come, and all I could do was count the breaths and the moans, picturing myself just going up and over the top of each one. One thing that I did use from all my hypnosis practice was saying "peace", picturing my belly and back more comfortable, but it was not a very peaceful-sounding "peace" at all…more like the sound of a dying cow, or Eric said the chorus of a death-metal song. I got in the shower again, and when I got out I noticed fluid running down my leg – finally my water had broken. We checked again and the cervix was entirely out of the way, there was no cord prolapse, and no feet presenting – everything was finally lined up right and I could birth this baby. Have to say I still didn't believe it would happen at all though. I still didn't have any strong urge to push, but the contractions were coming so fast, and finally it seemed that they just never stopped…and it seemed to feel a little better if I would bear down some at certain points, so I was doing that just for comfort.

I ended up on my hands and knees, sort of sitting back onto my heels to push for a while. I could feel her starting to move down, and at the peak of one push we saw meconium. Freaked me out for a minute thinking I was bleeding a lot or something, but Wendy assured me it was just meconium, totally expected for a breech birth, and I was actually encouraged that that meant we were getting somewhere. Wendy suggested that I could try squatting while hanging between Eric's legs as he sat on the bed. As soon as I got up into that position, the baby just rocketed down; I could feel her hit bottom. Within a couple of pushes we could see bottom, and I reached down and felt, and funnily my thought was "I guess this means it's too late to have a cesarean now". Then I felt her moving down more and my perineum stretching, and a bizarre sensation that she was spinning around or something. A few more pushes and the butt was mostly out…then on the next push I felt her legs come free, then arms, and Eric said "here's our baby sweetie, our baby is coming!" and I looked down and saw her lying below me, and then Wendy picked up her body and I felt her head roll out, and there she was! My baby! She was in my arms, slippery and new. I rubbed her back; she opened her eyes up but wasn't breathing just yet. Maryanne and Wendy were checking her heart tones, sucking some gunk out of her mouth, brought a bit of oxygen, and she pinked up quickly. Wendy said, "See, who says breech birth is such a big deal!" I just held her in awe talking to her and welcoming her, and Eric asked if it was a boy or a girl. I looked – girl! Just as Simon had predicted.

I felt a gush of blood and fluid, and Maryanne cut the cord and the placenta was born. I heard someone say, "Here's why she was breech!" There was a true knot in her umbilical cord, apparently pretty rare. I guess she knew what she was doing when she dug in her heels and refused to be flipped. I was thrilled to be able to really eat again and had several pieces of the pizza that had smelled so nauseating before. Simon came in to meet and kiss his new baby sister. A bit later we got in the bath together and it was magical just to be with her, enjoying her, getting to know her…and not on a morphine drip, no hole in my guts, nothing shoved down her throat, never taken from me. I had only a couple of little tears, no stitches. Eric, Lily, baby and I all slept together until morning, Mary made breakfast and took great care of us, and we headed home. Every bit of this harrowing, endless adventure had been incredibly worth it, and I'll never forget it.

Eva Robin

At 3:30 a.m. on September 2, 2002, I woke with a little leaking. I thought it might be amniotic fluid, but wasn't sure. There was a tiny bit of bloody mucus in the toilet, and a little pink when I wiped – turned out it was a bit of the mucus plug. I started to get excited – I had been saying I'd go into labor on Labor Day, and maybe this was it! I was 41 weeks and 1 day pregnant. I had a hard time going back to sleep, with excitement and mild contractions, not much different than I'd been getting for a few days. Randy stirred, and I told him what was going on and he said, "Are we having a baby today?" I finally fell asleep around 5:30 a.m., and woke again at 8:00 am. I continued to have mild contractions for the morning, but they were different – maybe more regular or noticeable or crampy. Around 9:00 a.m. I called the midwife, Merilynne, and gave her the update. I asked her "Am I going to have a baby today?" and she said to be patient, that these were all good signs that things were progressing, but it could be today, or it could be in the next few days. She said to call back between 3:00 – 5:00 p.m. with an update. So I tried to go about my morning like nothing was different, to normalize the day, so I didn't get my hopes up. Catherine called and I told her what was up, and assured her that it seemed like something was different, but it could still be a few days even.

Around 11:00 a.m., the contractions started getting more noticeable. I would stop and breathe through them. They were not too painful, but nothing to ignore either. Randy was cooking risotto in preparation for a BBQ that evening with Bill and Becky. But our friends cancelled, and so I encouraged him to bring them some. I went upstairs and tried to watch Law and Order reruns on cable, and rest. I could feel that the baby was posterior – I had been battling the posterior position for several days now. So I would lie on my side and push the butt toward the front of my belly, and then get on hand and knees for a while to let gravity help. I was determined not to have a posterior labor, and it worked. Once she settled into a more optimal position, the labor picked up, and I started having to vocalize a bit during contractions, which were occurring every 6-10 minutes. Things were intensifying quickly. Around 2:00 p.m., I was on my hands and knees in the hallway, vocalizing loudly during contractions. We called the midwife again. She asked if I wanted her to come over and be checked. I was having a hard time figuring out what I wanted. I didn't want to have a dilation check and be told I was only at 2 cm, so I equivocated. She asked to talk to Randy, and she heard me make my way through several contractions. She said he could get me in the pool for 20-30 minutes, but get me out if my contractions slowed down. I was also hesitant to have her come over because I was thinking I had a long way to go, and I was still trying to "normalize" a bit, and prepare for a long haul.

In the meantime, I was definitely working hard. I told Randy to call my mother and Catherine. He held the bucket for me as I threw up the plums and peaches I had eaten earlier. It was getting harder. He went to fill up the pool, but was having a hard time with the hose – the sink was shallow and he couldn't get the hose to fit tightly to the attachment. Poor Randy, he was really hurrying! I was in my bathroom alternating between the floor and the toilet, working very hard, not aware of time. Finally he got the pool filled up. It was a little hot, but it felt so good to get in. Randy would get the bucket for me when I needed to be sick, and I'd hold his forearms for contractions, and he'd put juice or water in front of me to sip. At some point, maybe around 4:00 p.m., he called the midwife again and said things were picking up and maybe she should come over. Actually, I think his words were "Julie's getting a bit more uncomfortable." I don't think he realized how close we were – he was also thinking we had a longer haul. Turns out we were in transition! I heard myself saying, "I can't do this Randy, I can't do it." I knew that's what women said in transition, but it all seemed so soon. It was all encompassing, and it took every bit of strength I had just to get through each contraction.

I rested well against the side of the pool in between contractions. At one point, I reached out of the pool – sending a cascade of water onto the floor, with Randy looking a bit forlorn. But mostly, I just went along for the ride. I didn't fight it, I wasn't afraid of it, but I was really feeling like I could not tolerate it any more. I started getting really hot, and Randy suggested getting out of the pool. I was on my hands and knees on the floor and then with a contraction, I heard my breathing change. I said "Randy I think I'm pushing!" He had great surprise in his voice, and said, "You're pushing?? Um, let's get you back in the pool!" He paged Merilynne again and left a voicemail that said I was pushing – that was about 4:15 p.m.

At some point, Mickey (the other midwife) called. It turns out she was on call because the only available apprentice was Amanda, who was just starting out and could only be a third attendee. I heard Randy on the phone with her, updating her on our progress. I didn't know Mickey was to be involved, and thought he was talking to my cousin and couldn't figure out why on earth he was talking on the phone while I was pushing and told him to get off the phone! Little did I know, Merilynne had paged her with our number as call-back, because when she got Randy's second message that I was pushing, she high-tailed it over, not wanting to wait for Mickey's call. Merilynne arrived around ten till five. Mickey and Amanda each came in soon thereafter. Someone checked me and said the head was most of the way through the birth canal already. She could feel it, and a bag of waters.

The presence of the midwives was wonderful. Suddenly there were these soothing women around, giving me encouragement and telling me how wonderful I was doing. Mickey had her face and lips on my shoulder and I'd lean into her, and her skin felt so good, as if restoring me between the pains. Her tender and gentle touches were so soothing. The voices of the midwives were incredibly grounding and reassuring – it makes me want to cry to think about it now. I remember someone putting my hair up better, out of my face. And I remember occasionally having to reposition myself so they could check the fetal heart rate with the Doppler, and we could all hear it. It slowed only once, when the baby was almost out. I remember someone lighting the candles, and I could smell them, and someone getting my camera and taking pictures. Randy was keeping cold wet washcloths on me, and he'd squeeze cold water over my head and shoulders between contractions, and it felt so good! During contractions, I'd get on my knees and hold his forearms and curl up and push. He'd encourage me, and his voice sounded so good.

The midwives told me it was Ok to push into the pain, and they'd let me know when to ease up. I started to feel the head come down during a contraction, and then recede back up in between. This happened a few times, and then I felt it come down and stay down. There was commotion, and excitement in the room. I know I said something about feeling burning at some point. And at some point the midwives told me to breathe through a contraction – not push. And then amongst the excitement and commotion and change in energy, I pushed and they saw the head and I pushed and pushed and then I felt her! I felt her slide out of me and it was the most incredible feeling in the world! Randy said she just shot out all at once, as soon as the head emerged. I had been on my left knee, holding onto Randy, with my right leg kind of raised to make room. I heard Randy's voice – the excitement in it, the laughter in it! And I flipped over and there was this little person, this little writhing, wiggling, warm, wet person placed quickly onto my chest and covered with blankets and a hat and it was my baby! Wow, we did it! Oh my gosh, this little person was inside me all this time and I didn't even know what she looked like! And I didn't know she was a she yet – I lifted her feet and looked and said "It's a girl!" and looked at Randy and he was smiling and laughing and so happy and I was crying I think and laughing and breathing and it was all such a miracle.

The midwives guided me to push out the placenta, which I did, though I really didn't feel a contraction or an urge to. They clamped the cord because it had stopped pulsing, and Randy cut it. At some point, he took the baby and I was helped out of the pool. I started shaking so hard, I couldn't control it – I was cold and weak. They wrapped me up and got me up the several steps to my bedroom, where I was to stay for the next several days. The little champ was nursing within thirty minutes of her birth, and remains a champion nurser. An herbal bath was prepared and I was helped into it – it felt great. And little Eva, our miracle, was given to me in the bath, to be soothed and healed as well. We had my first pee, a newborn exam, a perineum exam, and some post-partum instructions. Catherine came over and started crying – it was so good to see her! It had happened so fast nine hours total, she wasn't able to get here in time for the birth. But she stayed

with me, and helped me to and from the bathroom and did best friend things for

hours. Eventually, everyone left, and it was just I Randy and our little Eva –our

family – in our bed, holding and resting and nursing and napping and basking in

wonderment.

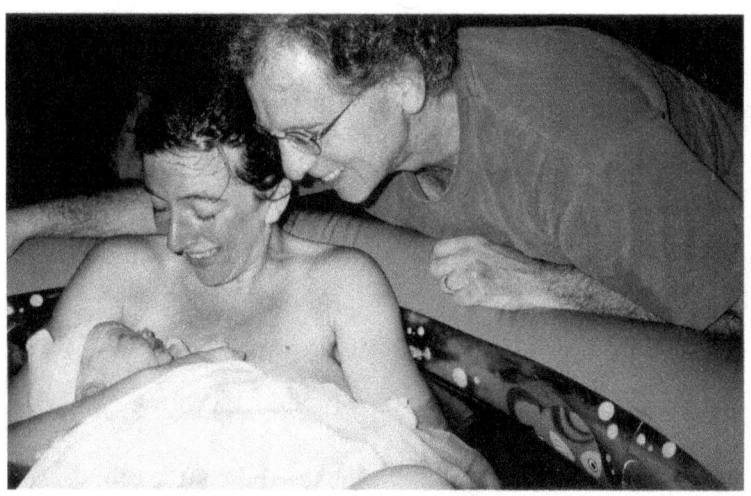

Mommy	:Julie
Daddy	:Randy
City State	:Ann Harbor, MI
Age at birth	33
Birth	:1
Baby's Name	:Eva Robin

Morgan Marie Coover

This is the story of Morgan and her unexpected arrival. We had been trying for a second baby shortly after our son, Brandon, had turned two. However, we hadn't been able to conceive. In April I was two weeks late with my period and I bought a pregnancy test and it was positive. We made an appointment with my OB/GYN and he confirmed the pregnancy.

Well, my pregnancy was relatively uneventful except for the morning sickness, which I did not have during my first pregnancy. At one of my last checkups the doctor was concerned that the baby may be too big to have a vaginal birth after cesarean. I had a sonogram and it confirmed that the baby might be well over nine pounds. My husband and I reluctantly agreed to a cesarean. (Recalling the experience we had had with our first.) We scheduled the surgery for December 16, 1997.

On Sunday, December 14, we awoke, got Brandon ready and ourselves ready for church. We went to church. Well, God must have had an impact on our little one's life because during the sermon I began having some real uncomfortable back pain. Randy rubbed my back and that eased my discomfort. After church, we took Brandon to Sunday school and we stood on the street talking to our minister and I finally told Randy that we better get to the hospital. The minister's daughter told us before we were leaving that we would have a baby before suppertime. Little did we know what God had planned for us.

We went home to call the doctor and to retrieve my bag. Upon entering the house my water broke, my husband was on the phone with the doctor and he heard the panic in my voice. He said to get to the hospital. It took me ten minutes to get to the car. We forgot our cell phone but remembered to make arrangements to have Brandon picked up. We were on our way down I-81 on the way to the hospital. The contractions were coming closer and closer together. I felt the baby move down and I said, "Oh no, the baby is coming!" Randy said, "what?" I barely heard him because at that very moment I was reclining the seat back, pulling down my pants and screaming at Randy to drive faster. We were passing truck drivers and I guess they probably couldn't see what was going on because they were angry at first that we were beeping at them.

We didn't make it to the hospital on time. Morgan Marie Coover arrived in the front seat of the family station wagon at 12:01 p.m., a half-hour after we left church. She weighed in at 8 pounds 15 ounces. Randy continued driving during the whole birthing process. Morgan had the cord wrapped around her neck, but after I removed it she left out a loud cry, and we wrapped her in my good leather coat for the remainder of the ten-minute journey to the hospital. They cut the cord outside the emergency room and I delivered the placenta in the delivery room.

The doctor came in about five minutes after we were up in labor and delivery. He said, "You sure went fast."

Mom	:Tina
Dad	:Randy
City State	:Carlisle, Pennsylvania
Age at birth	:31
Birth	:Second
Baby's name	:Morgan Marie
Baby's Height	:21 1/2" long;
Baby's Weight	:9lbs. 15 1/2 ozs.

Twin Homebirth After Cesarean

I guess it really begins with the birth of their older brother, my third child, born in 2001. I had planned a homebirth, as I had really hoped to avoid unnecessary hospital interventions. As things would turn out, I ended up transporting to the hospital and having an emergency cesarean due to transverse lie. Before his birth, we had wanted a large family one-day. I was so devastated by the loss of the birth I had planned. I was also overwhelmed by the fear that I would never again experience natural childbirth due to a prior cesarean. Because of that my husband and I decided we didn't want any more children.

Just last year, things shifted in our thinking a bit. I had researched vaginal birth after cesarean (VBAC) enough to know that it is a safe option in situations where induction, augmentation, and other interventions could be avoided. We decided to try to conceive our fourth child. After I was pregnant, I began my search for a provider. I found that several local hospitals (including the 3 closest to me) no longer allowed planned VBACs. None of the local doctors would be fully supportive of a VBAC. I looked into homebirth with a direct entry midwife. I learned that the midwife licensing board made it illegal for direct entry midwives to deliver VBACs in my state as of 2004 (even though they had successfully been attending VBAC homebirths for many years before then.) Only a CNM could deliver a VBAC at home, and no CNMs in my state could find a backup OB to support them in a VBAC homebirth.

Through referrals from our many friends who had given birth at home near us, we found a very naturally-minded CNM. She worked in a neighboring state but used to in our area before she moved to Tennessee (I live in SC). While she was not willing to drive all the way to SC (over 3 hours from her) while I was in labor, she was willing to take me on as a client provided we were willing to meet in Asheville, NC. This was two hours from me, and just over an hour from her. So we would drive there for appointments and for the birth. We agreed, and began our search for somewhere to stay for two weeks before and two weeks after our due date, so that we would already have a temporary home in Asheville to have our homebirth VBAC (HBAC).

A month after securing our midwife's services (just before our first appointment with her) and feeling confident with our course of action, we went in for a non-medical ultrasound to find out gender. We were shocked to learn that we would be having both a little girl and a little boy. The sonographer took several extra pictures for us including several showing that we had two placentas, which later proved valuable information. Later that day we panicked, calling our midwife and letting her know we would be finding an OB and switching providers. We were just too scared to go through with a twin HBAC.

We did a little more research, though, and found that twin VBAC moms are no more likely to suffer uterine rupture than singletons, and we learned that twins

with two placentas have minimal complications (if any) compared to singletons.
So we began to wonder if we should resign ourselves to a mandatory cesarean at
the hands of a surgeon. I called my midwife back and asked her what her
experience had been with twins. It turned out she has delivered tons of twins
when working in hospitals, and almost twenty sets of twins (including many twin
VBACs) since switching to a primarily home-based practice twelve years ago. All
twin births were successful; none required transport. We switched back to the
original plan, and began preparations for a twin HBAC.

Labor Begins:

For weeks I had been having strong and uncomfortable contractions-- so many
so that I was terrified of pre-term labor. Somehow I made it to 36 weeks (the
earliest my midwife would attend a twin homebirth) and we relocated to Asheville
NC. My husband stayed with the kids and me Fridays through Mondays, and he
went home every Monday to work a full week. In spite of regularly growing
contractions, I made it past 38 weeks, and when I was 38 weeks and 1 day
(measuring 50 cm), my husband went back home to work his week. That night, I
tossed and turned, having contractions in my sleep. Tuesday morning, May 8th,
around 3:30 a.m., I was awakened with painful contractions coming every two
minutes. This had happened before, so I tried all my usual tricks to make the
"false labor" go away. I had a glass of diluted wine, drank lots of water and lied

down, and around 4:15 a.m. I gave up and got into the bathtub to see if that calmed them. At 4:45 a.m., still unsure if I was in real labor or not, I called my husband and asked him to come be with me just in case it was time. At 5:00 a.m., I called my midwife and let her know what was going on. She told me to call my other labor assistants and get everyone on their way.

Around 5:30 a.m., as I was making the bed and getting my birth pool ready (I really wanted a water birth), my water broke and things intensified. Around 7:00 a.m., the midwife arrived and allowed me to get into the birth pool to take the edge off the contractions, and the water was so soothing! By 7:15 a.m., the midwife's assistant arrived, and by 7:30 a.m. my husband was there. Things get a little blurry after that point, since I was in a good bit of pain. At first, I did really well, breathing through the contractions, relaxing, and staying calm. By around 9:30 a.m., in transition, I was exhausted already, and begged to move to the bed so I could lie down.

The births:

Soon, I told my midwife I thought I might be feeling the urge to push with contractions, and that it actually made me feel a little better to push a tiny bit. So, with the next contraction, I began pushing. As things would turn out, I pushed a long time for a little baby who had spent the last two weeks at a +1 station. It didn't take long for him to crown, but then he couldn't make it any farther. It turns out that the OB who did my episiotomy with my second child has stitched me up more tightly than necessary, so I had to stretch really slowly like a first time birth. For over 15 minutes, I would have a contraction and his head would bulge, but not come out, and then I would spend the short break between the contractions in pain. I was worried crying about how this was affecting the baby, but my midwife checked his heart tones after each contraction and reassured me that as long as his heart rate was good, we were okay. Finally, with me lying on my side and yelling things like "get it out-- get this baby out of me!!" in a very non-relaxed and un-peaceful way, my sweet boy was born at 10:49 a.m. He was crying as soon as his head was out, and was nursing like a little barracuda 20 seconds after he was born! He pinked up right away, and they delayed clamping and cutting the cord until it had stopped pulsing.

We left him at the breast, since the nursing might stimulate contractions to get baby B into position, and from the time my boy was born until the time his sister's head was firmly engaged in the birth canal, my midwife's assistant held her in place from the outside so she wouldn't flip. After a few minutes, contractions started up again but they shortly became a little painful and I asked someone to take him so that he would be safer than I felt he was in my arms. I switched to using a breast pump between contractions to keep things going, and soon enough I knew it was time to push her out. I was exhausted, and not very enthusiastic about it at first, and couldn't bring myself to push that hard. I was expecting that after just birthing one baby, the second one would be easier, so I don't think I was expecting the challenge she became. At some point they moved me into a squatting position to push for a few contractions. It was so hard to support myself that once the baby's head was down into the canal; I was asking to lie back on the bed again. So, I pushed for the next several contractions propped up in a half-sitting position. She wasn't moving down very much, and I was getting discouraged. So I forced myself to get a little more energetic about the pushing (since that's what my body was telling me to do anyway). After several contractions, there wasn't a lot of progress, and I asked to get back on my side again. At that point, things started to move along, and after a very long pushing stage, my sweet little girl was born, posterior and forehead-first, with her cord wrapped around her shoulders, at 12:46 p.m. Her posterior position had contributed to my extended pushing phase and slow descent with her, and after her head was out I had to pant instead of push while they untangled her from her cord. She was a little slower to pink up, and took a little longer to figure out how to nurse, but soon enough was alert at my breast like her brother had been!

I birthed the placentas at 1:09 p.m., and although there were clearly two separate placentas, they had fused together in the middle and came out in one giant piece that likely weighed between 5 and 6 pounds-- almost like delivering a third baby, but without the giant head! I needed one stitch to fix a small tear from my daughter's difficult birth. I was bleeding heavily, and over the little while after the birth had one intravenous shot of pitocin and two shots in the hip. I was also given my first dose of methergine (which I will still be taking until 2 days postpartum), and given a lot of blood building and iron supplements to help replace what was being lost. After a while (I'm not sure how long) of still bleeding heavily, my midwife told me that she believed I had several clots just above my cervix that were preventing things from closing down properly. She said, "Well, you aren't going to like me very much for this, but I think the best course of action is for me to reach in." Apparently, excessive bleeding is a bit more common with twin pregnancies since my uterus had two raw areas from two placentas instead of just one.

Thoughts the next day:

So, I have now had my first completely unmedicated, natural birth, my first home birth, my first VBAC, and my first twin birth. What an experience! I feel so good about how it all happened, and I am so thankful that we chose the path we did because I know that I otherwise would have been forced into an unwanted, and completely unnecessary, cesarean. Although I worried a bit before the birth about the toll that being so big was going to take on my uterine scar, during labor I never once questioned how my scar was holding up. I have no regrets about my birth experience, for the first time ever, and feel only positive about how it all went down-- not exactly easy, but definitely uncomplicated.

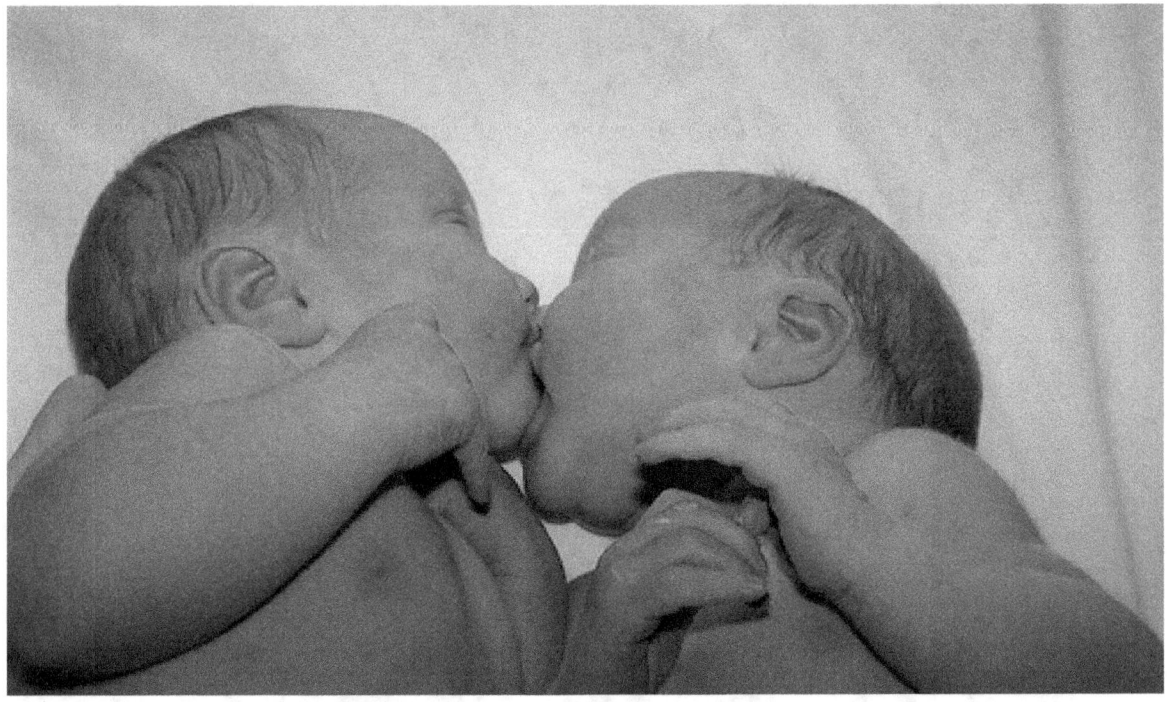

My babies were at the breast within minutes of being born, and my precious

husband was able to be more involved in this birth than any other-- what a

wonderful support he was! My other children were able to come in shortly after

each birth to see their new little siblings, and the babies' first night was spent

bonding with their parents and siblings, rather than being poked, prodded,

weighed, and messed with all night long. I've been able to rest when I need to,

recover in a way that feels best, and avoid being poked, prodded, and beeped to

death during an already exhausting and physically challenging time. I am SO

THANKFUL for these beautiful little babies, their curious little eyes, and their

sweet little cries. They are beautiful, precious, sweet, and fun to watch and be

with. What a blessing!

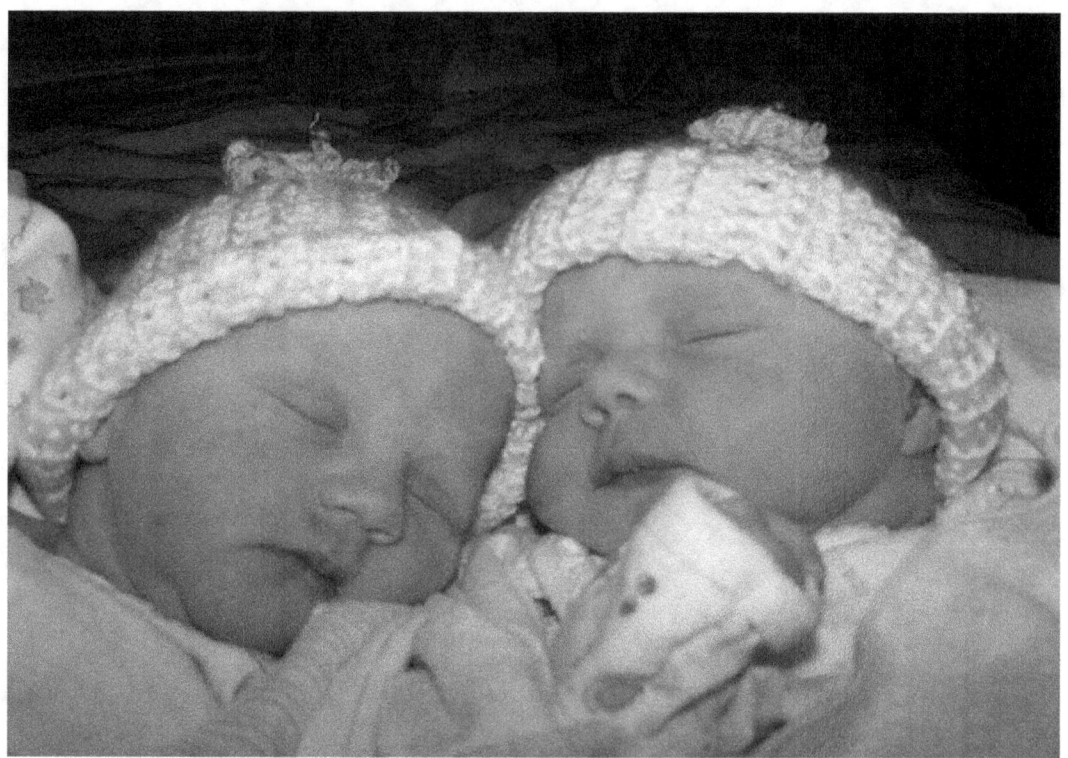

Solomon

I've always heard "Ask and you shall receive," but I now know that God truly has a sense of humor! Our son, Solomon, was due on September 6, 2003. That same day, my partner Kenyatta, Solomon's father, was celebrating his tattoo studio's 6-year anniversary. A party would take place that evening, full of music, many friends, family, and clientele, and lots of fun. But before the celebration, I was scheduled to get a massage from a friend of ours who specializes in all types of therapy. She worked on me for almost two hours, and I believe my contractions started in the midst of the massage. Prior to making the appointment, I had a feeling a massage would "get things moving" on the day our son was due.

Afterwards, we arrived to the studio ready to party! A friend that I ran into at the beginning of my pregnancy (who highly suggested that I purchase the book Birthing From Within), attended the party that evening. She also made the suggestion that I just enjoy myself and not get caught up in timing my contractions. Boy, what appropriate advice for me! I danced and danced and danced all night to good music that made me feel fine. When my contractions got stronger, I just closed my eyes and swayed back and forth to the music. At about midnight, September 7th, the contractions began to get stronger to the point that I had to sit down. Three girlfriends, whom I called my personal doulas, lovingly cared for me; one rubbed my feet, one massaged my hands and the other placed cold cloths around my neck.

With my son's godmother organizing our departure by lining our car with plastic on my seat, Kenyatta and I were off to go…home. I did not realize I was in active labor, so I just wanted to go home and get some rest. Even with my contractions increasing in strength and discomfort, we, in fact, passed the hospital on the way home. Once we arrived to the house, I asked Kenyatta to run a bath with lavender for me (I was hooked on lavender's aroma during my pregnancy!). Little did I remember from class that to slow down contractions in early labor you take a bath. In active labor, taking a bath speeds up the process. Again, unbeknownst to me I was in active labor. So ten minutes out of the tub, after closing my eyes for only ten seconds, I'm on the bed ready to push.

Kenyatta and I immediately performed our co-chanting, a technique we learned from our Birthing In Awareness class, by saying in unison, "OPEN!" It was time! I told Kenyatta to wake my mother and let her know her third grandson was on his way. When she arrived in the room, she said, "Um Kim, I don't know if we should do this here." I replied with, "Just let it flow, Mommy. Just let it flow." My mother left to call the paramedics, but Solomon and I were in no mood to wait. From lying on my side, I instinctively got on all fours and began to push. Three or four good pushes did the trick. Kenyatta was on the phone with Solomon's godmother and yelled, "I see the head!" Then, in Kimberly "the coordinator" fashion, I yelled, "Get the camera!" I took hold of Solomon's head and with one final push guided him out. The paramedics arrived a few minutes later.

Now, from a chronological perspective, Kenyatta and I desired natural birth; to welcome our baby into the world without any outside manipulation. A friend of ours informed us of local doulas' classes called Birthing In Awareness (actually based on the suggested book mentioned above). I am 99.9% certain that this 6-week course prepared us for the amazing birth we were to experience. This class was greatly a reminder that if we "let our bodies give birth," and truly listen to our intuition, we could have the natural childbirth we desired. I believe one of the class exercises specifically prepared us for this awesome birth. We had to create a living birth plan, as opposed to just a written plan for the hospital file. The living birth plan is a collage on poster board, filled with words and images of the things we desired for our birth. This way, regardless who would be on staff at the hospital, from the doctors and nurses to housekeeping personnel, anyone that walked into my room would be able to see what I did and did not want for the birth. But beyond this objective, I believe that by completing the exercise, we were making a special prayer of what our hearts truly desired. Some of the plan's items read, "Do Not Speak/Offer Medication!" "The pain is strong, but you are STRONGER!" "Negative energy = Step Outside!" Everything we put on our living birth plan, we got…just in a different kind of way. The music, the people, even the lavender was all a part of the experience. More interesting to note is that the same picture of my grandmother, which was the focal point on the poster board, was on the dresser in the room where Solomon was born. Coincidence, I think not!

Because of my birth experience, I am becoming a certified doula (a woman that helps another woman). I would love to encourage and assist women to be confident in giving birth and to reassure them that they have all the "internal tools" they need to have the birth they want. I would give birth at home again in a heartbeat, for what better way to guarantee the personal "comforts of home!"

Mom	: Kimberly
Dad	: Kenyatta
City State	: Atlanta, Georgia
Age at birth	: 26
Birth	: First
Baby's Name	: Solomon
Baby's Weight	: 7lbs.

Laurel Anne

Background: My cesarean birth:

With my firstborn I planned a birth center birth with CNMs. I worked throughout my pregnancy (a mostly-desk job), walked a few times a week, followed the Brewer diet, took Bradley childbirth classes, saw a chiropractor, and thought I was doing everything I could to have a successful birth. At the end of my pregnancy I developed pitting edema to my knees (35 weeks) and my blood pressure started to rise at 39 weeks. Two days before my due date I woke up with a small amniotic leak, and when labor did not start within 24 hours, I took castor oil as suggested by the midwives. Labor finally started about 18 hours after the castor oil, in the middle of the night. The next morning, 48 hours after the amniotic leak, not knowing my blood pressure status, the CNMs advised by phone that I not be active while I was still laboring at home. In the afternoon we arrived at the birth center at 4 cm, and after 5 hours hadn't made any progress. My blood pressure was fine and I was up walking, in the shower, etc. They suggested Demerol to help me relax more fully, and when I didn't make progress after two hours "sleeping" under its influence, we transferred to the hospital for AROM, pitocin, and an epidural. After about 8 hours at the hospital and 25 hours of total labor, my temperature began to rise and the baby's heartbeat rose, signaling infection (or maybe just an epidural fever). It was decided that we needed to have a cesarean. The worst part of the entire experience was the 4 hours after the surgery, separated from my new son who was in the NICU. My exhausted husband shuttled between us as our family, doula, and midwife left us before he was released.

I had a period of mild depression for about 4 months after that experience, and immediately began reading about and planning a VBAC. Before I even became pregnant again, I decided that I would have a homebirth, and that I wouldn't be deterred. Amazingly, my husband's first reaction to this choice was positive, which was a huge relief.

The HBAC pregnancy:

I was active with my son age 2 and niece age 3, walking almost daily, eating a low-glycemic index and mostly organic diet, and using some herbs and supplements. I chose a lay midwife who made me feel entirely responsible for my baby's health, and myself and began seeking out homebirth, VBAC, and general birth groups for support. My background as a biologist and doula had built up a great deal of mental knowledge of birth, statistics, etc, and I knew that knowledge alone had not helped me in my first birth. Instead of reading technical birth preparation books, I read extensively things that helped me to trust birth and to work through my emotional issues and fears. I devoured birth stories, especially HBAC stories. For me it was key to find a way to listen to my instincts and my body. Even this reading I limited to the waning phase of the moon. As the moon waxed, I tried to focus on enjoying being pregnant and connecting with the baby. At about 6 months a pregnant friend and I did a cleansing ceremony where we read to each other the negative things about our previous births and then burned the lists, smudged each other, and finally shared our hopes for our upcoming births.

The HBAC Birth Story:

The weekend before the birth story begins I had cleaned my house thoroughly (about 4 hours of work) to host a homebirth meet up on Saturday, and then on Sunday went to my mother in law's for a tea in my honor (sort of a shower). People at both events noticed that I had "dropped" and a midwife friend even looked me over closely and said, "I know you're not due for 2 1/2 weeks...but I don't think you'll last that long!" The baby was born at 38 weeks and 3 days.

My labor began about 2:00 a.m. on a Thursday night, under a full moon, with small crampy contractions every 2-3 minutes. I was able to sleep until 8:00 a.m., but the contractions were still coming every 3 minutes, lasting just 20-30 seconds, and still very mild. I went about my normal routine, making breakfast for my son who is age 2 1/2. I called my midwife at about 9:00 a.m. and told her what was going on, she thought they were just "tune-ups" and that I should get some wine in case I needed it to help me sleep that evening (HA!). When my husband came downstairs at 10:00 a.m., he found me leaning on the counter, breathing slowly. I told him he wouldn't be going to work, the contractions were picking up. He went to tell work he wouldn't be in, and I continued to try to act normal--doing dishes, eating a half-cup of plain yogurt. When he returned about 10:45 a.m. both my son and I were a little frantic. I had to blow through contractions, even feeling trembly at the heights, and my poor son didn't understand why I wouldn't look at him or talk to him during these frequent episodes. So, I escaped to my shower, leaving instructions for my husband to call both my midwife and than his mother to come pick up our son.

While I was in the shower I talked to my midwife twice on the phone and she assessed my contractions. They were two minutes apart and 40 seconds long, and she said she'd be there in a couple of hours. I got out of the shower, leaving my long hair in a tangle on top of my head. I put on one of my favorite old sleep t-shirts and underwear, and lay down on my side in bed. By this time (about noon) my husband was able to help and I had him squeeze the fronts of my thighs between contractions, to alleviate the aching.

About an hour later I was kneeling leaning over my birth ball when our midwife's assistant arrived, and she checked the baby's heart rate (great), and jumped in to help my husband do hip squeezes. A little later, when my midwife arrived, I was up pacing the hallway. As my midwife and her assistant set up their things in my bedroom, my husband and I walked around. I would hang on to him or lean onto a wall during the contractions, which by this time were two minutes apart and lasting a minute or longer...not much downtime in between.

We also climbed up and down the stairs (between contractions), and I spent a longer than necessary time on the toilet, where I found bloody show/mucus plug about 3:00 p.m., and began to feel pushy at the height of contractions.

About 3:30 p.m. I asked my midwife to check me, as I said, "I want to push...I want it to be time to push"...of course it wasn't yet. I was 5 cm dilated (but stretching to 7 during contractions), 75% effaced and the baby was still high. Somebody said, "Soon you'll be able to nurse that baby!" and it really struck me...I remember repeating "nurse the baby" to myself a few times, almost in wonder, reminded that's why we were doing this. So my midwife began suggesting positions for me to try. First, lunging with my left foot up on my bed (mid thigh height), hip rotated out 90 degrees. I hung on to my husband and we lunged during the contractions, which definitely made the contractions more intense. It was at this point that I started growling, even roaring, through every contraction (and did this until the birth...I was hoarse the next day).

Then I climbed the stairs during contractions. This was when I got the most verbal support from my team--it must have looked and sounded like hard work! My husband even got the video camera to capture my otherworldly vocalizations. I went down and back up three times (2X more than everyone expected, I heard later) and then spent some time hanging on to the stair-rail in a squat. And then I hung over my birth ball again, but doing pelvic tilts and belly-dance-like hip rolls through the contractions. Trying to do the pelvic tilts was the most painful part of the entire birth...everything else I'd just call intense. At this point, about 5:30 p.m., my midwife checked me again and found I was 8 cm dilated, and the baby still needed to rotate more anterior and was still high. So, back to lunging, and sitting on the toilet with my left leg elevated, and lunging again.

Then I squatted at the end of my bed, deeply in that labor land/intuitive movement place. I would drop down during contractions and stand back up between. I really began to feel pushy at this point, and my midwife suggested that I try to break my own water with my finger. I could feel it, but I couldn't really concentrate during a contraction enough to do it. (It was a great suggestion, though.) I spent a bit more time in a squat, rolling my hips during contractions (as if I were going to try to walk in a squat position). Then my midwife gave me the go-ahead to push when I felt a very strong urge, and I did that for a while. My water broke. With the next contraction, my midwife said my cervix "melted away" and I was complete. After that I began to push in earnest--three or four 3-5 second pushes with each contraction, which were still coming every two minutes. At one point my midwife suggested I check to see where the baby was, and I found she was only in as deep as the second knuckle on my middle finger...so close!

When the baby began to crown, I felt only momentary burning, and then her head was out. I had to hold off pushing for a contraction as my midwife worked off a loop of cord, found a hand at her ear, and suctioned the baby. The last push was the best...that last slippery gush of baby and fluid...and it was done! She was born at 7:04 p.m.

We moved up on to the bed with the baby, and waited for the placenta for about half an hour. Laurel latched on, and I felt just a couple of contractions just before the placenta emerged with one little push. Upon inspection it was whole and healthy (I was still sort of worried something would go wrong and spoil the peace of our experience thus far). My midwife found I had two small 1st degree tears--one lateral (where her hand was at her ear) and one perineal. Neither needed stitches. Laurel Anne was 7lb 3oz and 21 inches long, exactly like me at birth! With big blue eyes and a healthy dose of dark brown hair; such a joy!

Mom	: Erin
Birth	: Second
Baby's name	: Laurel Anne
Baby's Height	: 21 inches
Baby's weight	: 7lbs 3oz

Aurora

I was sent home around 6:00 pm because my nurse thought I was having false labor. My contractions got more intense every minute and before long I was waddling around the room because it hurt to lie down. This was my first child, so I still wasn't sure if I was really having a baby or not yet. So, I drew a warm bath and tried to relax a bit in it. That must have relaxed all of my muscles because before I knew it, I was pushing! I gave a couple hard pushes and I felt a tiny bit of hair on a head starting to poke out. Right after that, the light went out in the bathroom, so I was alone in the dark around two in the morning having my baby! A couple more hard pushes and her head came out. One more and the baby was officially born! I grabbed her right before she would have hit the end of the tub and held her upside down to let the fluid drain from her lungs until I heard her breath on her own. I held her near my chest and felt to see it was a girl (my baby was born and I STILL hadn't seen her face!) A few minutes later the light came back on when it cooled down again (Old wiring).

I got to know Aurora for maybe ten minutes before I wrapped her up in every single towel I had in the bathroom (with her placenta) and placed her comfortably in front of the bathroom heater while I rinsed off.

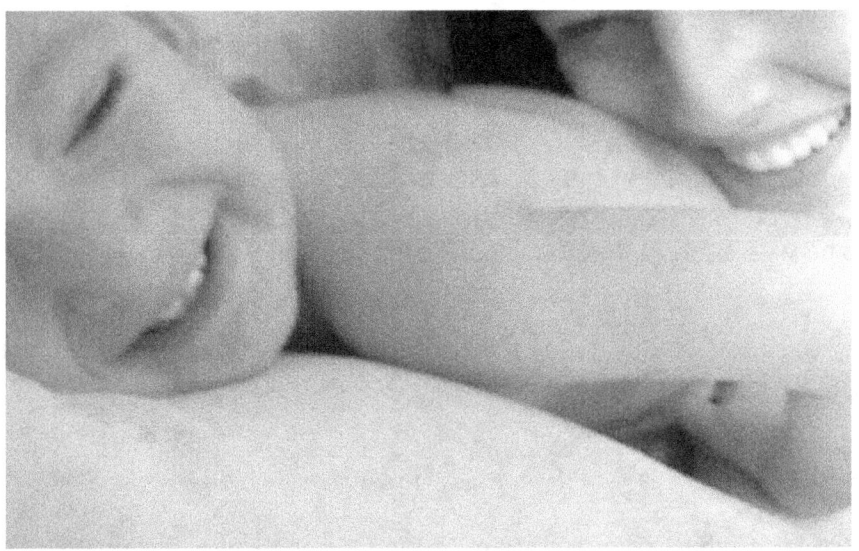

Mom	: Kara Nicole Groth
Dad	: James Douglas Riley
City State	: Springfield, Missouri
Age at birth	: 19
Birth	: First
Baby's name	: Aurora Lynn
Baby's Height	: 20 1/2 inches
Baby's Weight	: 7lbs. 6oz

ChristoFinn

I had a wonderful, incredible pregnancy with my son. We had a powerful connection while he was in utero that I was able to strengthen with yoga, meditation, and walks in the woods. During our "communications" my son guided me to the way he'd prefer to be born -- alone with only my husband, Graeme and me. I can truly attest that this was his idea, as it's something I had never contemplated before becoming pregnant. Many times throughout my pregnancy, I thought I was absolutely crazy to even consider having unassisted childbirth, but my son proved to be a very persuasive soul, convincing not only me, but also my reluctant husband. Whenever my confidence floundered I would repeat a line I had heard in a movie, "Faith is believing in something even when common sense tells you not to," and I would find comfort.

I found my journey to unassisted childbirth to be the most powerful, freeing, and empowering experience that I have ever had. Once I committed myself fully to free birthing my son, I learned his name in a dream. I had asked him one night before I went to bed to tell me what he'd liked to be named when he came earth side and all night I heard "ChristoFinn, ChristoFinn, ChristoFinn" whispered in my ear and saw the name printed out on a chalkboard that said "Finn for short." It was so vivid it woke me up and I was absolutely giddy. I told Graeme the next day and we smiled at each other. Although we'd never heard the name before, it seemed strangely familiar.

I spent the rest of my pregnancy getting in my best emotional and physical shape. I dedicated myself to my daily meditations and gentle yoga sessions. I also wrote frequently in my journal to help alleviate any fears, worries, or self-doubt. I wrote a list of 24 "Belief Statements" about my impending labor that I would read daily, among them that "My baby and I are fully deserving and capable of a gentle, blissful, and pain-free birth," and "My baby will come out healthy, breathing, and maybe even smiling."

When it came time to birth my baby, I felt ready. The only sign I had of impending labor was a dream the previous night of a newspaper heading reading "IT'S TIME!" And indeed it was. I woke up at 7:00 a.m. that morning to what I thought might be gas bubbles. But after I went to the bathroom and my "bubbles" still hadn't dissipated, I started thinking differently. When Graeme awoke I told him I didn't think I wanted him to go to his clients' houses that day and he looked at me expectantly and said "Really?" We were both very excited.

I ate a healthy breakfast and Graeme helped me pick up the house. Around 9:30 a.m. my contractions were getting too strong to ignore -- Graeme and I were both sure this baby would be there by noon. One of my belief statements was that I would have a short, effective labor of only 5-7 hours, so that's what I had myself geared up for. Graeme and I were having a lot of fun joking and laughing. We made love and it was incredibly intense and sensual. I was thinking that this labor-childbirth-thing was a piece of cake!

I set myself up in the bathroom because I knew that's where I'd feel the most comfortable. Graeme was right there with me rubbing my back and trying to make me laugh. My contractions, however, didn't seem to have any rhyme or reason to them. They all seemed strong, but they weren't getting any closer together. At times, they seemed to be getting further apart. Five hours went by, and then seven. I was already exhausted and realized I had closed myself off by giving my labor a deadline. Once seven hours passed I stopped keeping track.

It was also around then that I noticed I would have the best contractions whenever Graeme would leave the room. We both realized this and reasoned that he was actually doing too good a job of relaxing me. He would breathe with me through my contractions, and be very gentle and loving with his touch, but it seemed to be slowing me down. I told him then that I wanted to try laboring on my own for a while and he agreed.

Graeme (who really had been very reluctant about free birthing) surprised himself by remaining amazingly calm and peaceful throughout my labor. He let me labor alone while he watched movies, worked on his website, and even took a couple of naps. He would check on me frequently, but it was obvious to both of us that I was making more progress on my own.

I had moved to the toilet to labor, thinking this was the most natural position to relax my muscles and open myself up. My contractions kept building in strength, but I really couldn't tell how effective they were. I had long ago stopped keeping track of the time, but I noticed that it had gotten dark outside. Soon the only light I had in the bathroom were the three candles I had lit and a small stain-glassed turtle lamp (I had discovered after recovering from my second miscarriage that Turtles were a potent symbol of Motherhood and Protection, and I had decorated my bathroom with turtles to prepare for this birth).

I was getting very tired and at times frustrated. I kept thinking I had some psychological block that was keeping me from birthing my baby. I simply tried letting everything go with my breath. While I wouldn't say my contractions were painful, I also wouldn't say they were just "intense sensations that required my whole attention" as I'd heard before. And they weren't anywhere near "blissful" as I'd been hoping. They were strong and they were very tiring. I tried lying down on the bathroom floor a couple of times when I so badly needed a break, but that position didn't work for me at all. The only way I felt comfortable was on the toilet, so on the toilet I stayed, sighing loud and low with each contraction. When the contractions would prove to be too much and too close together, I'd ask the Universe for a break "even if it meant delaying labor" and I would get a much-needed respite.

I remember at one point being intensely thankful that I didn't have a midwife or doctor with me, because even though I wasn't keeping track of the time, I knew I must be taking long enough that a "professional" would most likely suggest something to "speed things up." I was so grateful there was no one there monitoring me or subconsciously pressuring me.

I alternated between too hot and too cold, and even though I was sweating I was also shivering. I had a baby blanket over my lap that I kept removing and replacing. I couldn't eat anything except a few grapes but I made sure to drink water after each intense contraction and I know that helped a lot.

Eventually my strong and tiring contractions gave way to something different -- overwhelming, body-rocking contractions that made my body involuntarily push. WOW! This was incredible! My breathing became louder and lower as I felt all the energy of the universe coursing through my body. Now we were getting somewhere! This was a welcome change from my other contractions, because even though they were more powerful, I could tell how effective they were. I can indeed say that these awe-inspiring contractions felt wonderful!

Graeme checked in on me as he had heard my breathing change and I said to him "It's getting so close." He must have checked in on me ten more times and each time I said the same thing "It's getting so close." After probably two hours of "it's getting so close" I said to myself "It's time to be a momma to this baby. Get him out!" I repeated that a couple of times and I could feel my baby move down. As I felt him moving down I said "Okay, baby, when I feel you crowning I'm getting off the toilet."

And then he started crowning. I immediately got off the toilet into a kneeling position. As his head started coming out I felt a burn strong enough to make me catch my breath, but it wasn't a "ring of fire" by any means. I grabbed the towel rack with the next contraction and subsequently pulled it out of the wall. Ah, the power of birth! My husband came in when he heard the crash and I announced "He's coming out!" Graeme offered to hold me up but I told him I was fine, so he sat down next to me and just watched.

I reached down and to my surprise I could feel my baby's head. It was soft and wet and wonderful! "I can feel his head!" I laughed and my baby wiggled which made me laugh some more. I gave a push and he came out a bit more, I touched him again and again there was wiggling and laughter. I then said "Okay, baby, time to get you out!" I pushed and immediately felt him coming out, "do you want to catch him?" I asked Graeme, but he wasn't fast enough and my baby landed softly in a pile of blankets just an inch below me.

He immediately started crying (in keeping with our deal to let me know he was breathing). I picked him up and laughed, "It's a boy! It's ChristoFinn!" Graeme beamed at me and agreed, "It is ChristoFinn." I laid him gently on my forearm so he could drain anything that might need draining and then put him to my chest. Our whole bathroom was lit up in magic. "We did it!" I kept exclaiming and laughing, "We did it." Our baby had stopped crying and was looking around, and then my husband saw it first, Finn smiled at us. This would be a perfect place to end his birth story, but there's so much more.

I thought our baby would be there before noon; instead Finn was born two minutes before midnight. And I wouldn't have had it any other way. I learned so much more about myself in a 17-hour labor, than I most likely would have in a 7-hour labor. Graeme asked to take pictures directly after the birth and of course I said yes. He took wonderful pictures of us, me still kneeling with Finn to my chest, covered in blood and birth. It was beauty in its most raw and perfect state. Graeme said he'd never seen me look like that before, like a goddess-- a Turtle Goddess. He tells people my eyes have been changed forever.

The placenta still hadn't come out, but we decided to move to the bedroom where we'd all be more comfortable, so we maneuvered very carefully to a new spot on the bedroom floor. There we just sat and stared at this new, beautiful being, whose eyes were too wide and alert for a newborn. Finn didn't want to nurse; he just wanted to stare at us as much as we wanted to stare at him. I'll never forget our first bonding.

Two hours later, the placenta still showed no signs of coming out but we were ready to cut the cord. It had long ago stopped pulsing so we asked Finn's permission to cut it. We believe he said it was fine, so we did. There was a bit of blood but he didn't seem bothered by it. I really wanted the placenta out, but didn't welcome the thought of any more contractions, so I squatted over a bowl and pinched my nipple very hard and whoosh! Out it came in one fell swoop!

Who-hoo, I was free! I cut off tiny bits of the placenta and swallowed them whole, knowing this would help me heal. Then the three of us -- a new family-- worked our way to the kitchen where we had the best meal of pancakes and bacon. Food had never tasted so good!

The next three days we were all on an incredible natural high. Everything was steeped in magic as if we'd entered another dimension. Our bonding had been so intense that it was impossible to tell where one of us ended and the other began. I would look in the mirror and see Finn's image. Graeme would look at his hands and see his son's hands. When I dreamed, I dreamed Finn's dreams in black and white. We slept, ate, and breathed one another. If I could relive those first few days over and over again, oh, I would.

While our birthing experience was perfect and wonderful, I would be doing birthing women a disservice if I didn't mention my difficult recovery. As prepared as I was for birth, I was totally unprepared for how I would feel afterwards. I'd read too many accounts of how women rarely tear during unassisted childbirth, and how recovery was usually so much faster, that I didn't honor how much time *my* body would need to heal.

I literally had to crawl up and down the stairs for two days. Putting on pajama bottoms was challenging and I desperately wished for a nightgown. It didn't burn when I urinated, so I falsely assumed that my perineum had stayed intact, and I didn't take it as easy as I should have. Still, I started to gradually feel better every day so I started doing more and more.

Four weeks postpartum I started taking Finn on long walks. Five weeks postpartum I started running. I didn't think this was unreasonable as I heard stories of women returning to the gym within a week of childbirth, and of course I'd read those stories of tribal women going to work in the fields twenty minutes after giving birth. But this level of activity was unreasonable for me. I'd bleed a bit after a day of too much activity which would make me take a week off or so. But then I would resume and it became a continuous cycle, until at four months postpartum I could barely walk, or even sit without being in incredible pain.

I swallowed my pride and went to see my midwife (who I had stopped seeing midway through my pregnancy after I informed her of my plan to birth unassisted). It turns out I had a second degree tear that had started healing nicely by itself, until I started doing too much too soon. Ironically, my midwife said, "You listened to those stories of women going to the fields twenty minutes after birth didn't you? Well, what they don't tell you is that those are the women who hemorrhage and have the most difficulties." I was humbled. She sealed me up with silver nitrate -- which is not a fun procedure in the least! -- But thankfully, it did the trick.

In retrospect, I think I most likely tore after my baby had crowned. I was so anxious to get him out the rest of the way, that I think I rushed my body. I have no regrets, though, as it's all been a learning experience.

Incidentally, 21 out of my 24 "Belief Statements" came true. The three that didn't were all time-related -- how long my labor would be, how long it would take my placenta to deliver, and how long it would take me to recover-- teaching me that the concept of time doesn't matter in the whole big, beautiful scheme of things. ChristoFinn teaches this to me every day as I cherish each moment we spend together....

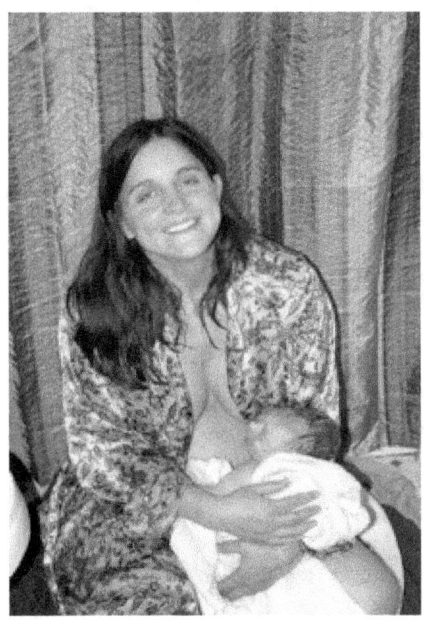

Mom	: Kate Street
Daddy	: Graeme Street
City State	: Essex, CT
Age at birth	: 34 years old
Birth	: First
Baby's name	: Chistofinn
Baby's Weight: 8 lbs.	

Violet

I feel this birth story cannot be fully understood unless you know about the birth of my first child, a beautiful, spirited boy, Gabriel Kelly. I was naive and uneducated about birth; I had no clue that there were any options other than having an obstetrician in a hospital. My 18 hour labor started early one morning with my water breaking at home. I got right to the hospital where I was laid in bed, subjected to at least 42 cervical checks (I lost count), along with every single intervention that they could present. Including an epidural that did not work properly causing me to shake violently. This all culminating in a very traumatic 'emergency' Cesarean Section for failure to progress/fetal distress. The spinal was placed 'too high' and I could not feel my lungs breathing for the entire operation. I suffered in silence from Post Traumatic Stress Disorder and Postpartum Depression in the months following, nobody knowing the true depth of my sorrow. In August of 2006, my husband mentioned having another child someday; I agreed to consider it on the condition that I would not have another Cesarean Section.

In the months following, I delved in to research, reading anything and everything having to do with all things birth, I did little else in those months but read about birth, talk about birth and breastfeed Gabriel. I wanted to be fully prepared to ask or answer any questions I had to. I read all of my mother's nursing books; she had just gotten her RN degree that very same year, so they were accessible. I realized all of the things I could/should have done differently in order to get the natural, joyful birth I had desired. Afterwards, I wrote my Lamentation of Birth, Gabriel's birth story. I attended a few local <u>International Cesarean Awareness Network (ICAN)</u> meetings. I joined their email list under the advice of a local homebirth midwife who had a Cesarean Section herself. Soon after I joined ICAN as a subscriber. Ross and I decided after all our research and revelations we would be happiest and safest having an unassisted birth at home when we got pregnant again. In November of 2006 we did just that, unbeknownst to us... well, more bluntly, our condom broke. I continued breastfeeding Gabriel until about April when he weaned himself, much to my dismay, because I so loved our nursing relationship. I had not wanted to conceive until Gabriel was at least two years old, but the universe had other plans I guess.

All in all, my pregnancy was very healthy and happy. I was active and very excited to have another baby coming. I did my own prenatal care, even checking the baby's heart rate from time to time with a stethoscope. I borrowed one from my mother. Except one prenatal visit to an obstetrician to get 'proof of pregnancy' in case I needed it for a birth certificate or something. I continued learning all I could about birth all the while forming my own ideas and ideals; making it my own, so to speak.

My labor started very slowly and lightly with irregular, weak contractions on Friday night August 17th, my sister was over for the weekend and we took her home on Saturday evening. The whole hour and a half drive out to my parents home I was having 'secret' contractions every few minutes, because we were keeping my family in the dark about our birth plans so as not to cause needless conflict and stress, so I could gestate in peace. On our way home, I knew I wanted to have this baby soon, so we decided to go to the mall and walk around for a few hours.

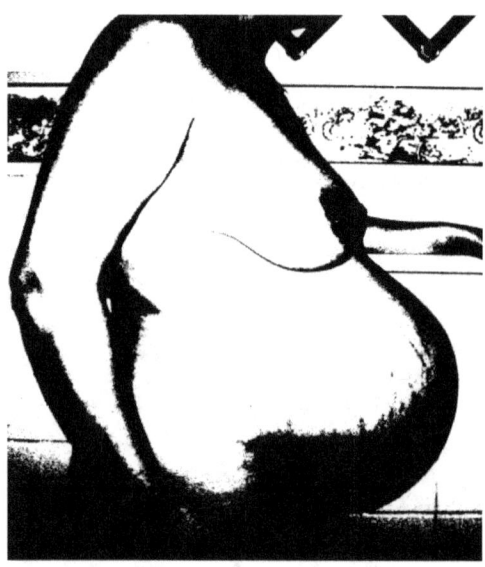

On Sunday August 19th when it came time for Ross to get ready for work at about 9:00 p.m. we were not sure if he should go in or not. So I asked him to check my cervix, I was open to 6 cm, so we figured he could call in to work and stay with me, get the birth tub ready and get Gabriel in to bed. Ross made me some wild rice soup because I figured I was in for a long night and I would be hungry, by the time I finished the bowl I was ready to get in the tub and relax, I must have been waiting for Gabriel to be sleeping for labor to really pick up.

In the tub, I was moving around constantly in slow voluptuous movements; I was never still during a contraction. If Ross laid his hands on me in any way, even if it was very gently or lightly, I felt as if I was put in a cage and I would panic causing the contraction to hurt rather than just take focus. I needed complete control over any touching, so I touched him when I needed contact, but he had to keep his hands off.

An hour or two later, I must have been in transition; I was in and out of the tub every other contraction because nothing felt 'right' for very long; I thought to myself, 'I must be in transition; I am acting like an animal right now!' Finally, I chose to make a little nest of pillows on the mattress we had put on the floor in front of our couch. I was leaning on the couch and on my pillows in between contractions. I was rising up like a wave and either kneeling or squatting down deeply for contractions. All of my thoughts at this point were 'soft and round', like a woman.

After a while I started sleeping between contractions, which was so nice because I was beat, and my sleepiness must have been catchy because I looked up at Ross who was sitting on the couch and he was sleeping too! At this point the 'pain' was very intermittent (when a contraction would 'sneak up' on me, it hurt more), and mostly located in the tops of my thighs and sometimes in my hips. Suddenly starting at the base of my skull and moving down like a wave, my body started pushing; it was a very strange sensation, kind of hot, dizzy and tingling like being tipsy. I looked up at Ross quizzically and said, "I'm pushing?" He gently replied "I know, it's okay if that's what your body has to do." I taught him well, I think. I had been so determined not to consciously push at all, to just 'go with the flow' so to speak, and that is what happened, I made sure not to think about it too much.

My water broke with a loud pop during a contraction I was rolling my hips through. After the contraction I compulsively looked down at the sheets to make sure the water was clear, it was, and I wondered why I looked, I knew it was fine. I continued rocking, rolling my hips, rising and falling and pushing when the need struck. I liked when my body pushed, it (and I) felt so ethereal, so powerful and Devine, yet very primal at the same time.

I kept this up for a while watching the trees sway back and forth in rhythm with me, mirroring the ebb and flow of my body, suddenly I was compelled to tell Ross "If you're going to catch this baby, you better get back there." I guess I did not want him jumping behind me abruptly and shaking the bed when I needed concentration and stillness. I reached inside of myself to see what I could feel, and I swore I was touching a tiny butt cheek. I asked Ross what he could see, the baby was just centimeters from crowning and he could not see anything. After a few more contractions (they seemed very far apart, who knows how long it really was), I asked Ross "What is it?" (Meaning a butt or a head, obviously I knew it was a baby) he said nothing for a long time because he could not tell what it was, aside from a wrinkly wet 'thing', and he wisely avoided saying "I don't know" knowing intuitively a reply like that would not be received very well at all. Very soon though, he saw it had hair, and told me so. I was a little relieved, although I was totally comfortable being at home by ourselves if the baby had been breech, I was just so sure that the baby was in the LOA position and I honestly would have been a little annoyed if I had been wrong.

Out of nowhere it felt like Ross was pulling my labia apart to get a better look, I said, "Don't touch, don't touch it!" He was not touching me at all, although he did not say anything back, I got the impression the intense stinging was not going to stop, and was the baby's head, not Ross' hands. I got scared at that point, the fact that a baby was coming out of my vagina somehow snuck up on me, and the sting got way worse. I will probably always wonder if it was the head stretching me open more, the fact that I was scared, or both. With the next push Ross said the head was out, and then said, "Hang on honey, the cord's wrapped." Now, in my head I was screaming 'No, no, no, that feels wrong, stop touching, please.' But, I actually said, very calmly and sweetly, "Don't worry, just unwrap it when the baby's out." I felt the baby turn to let the shoulder out, and the baby slid out into Ross' hands on the bed. The stinging was instantly gone, and I turned around and held my screaming, bright pink baby so close, I said, "Hi, oh my baby, I love you so much, I'm your mama, I love you! Hi there, oh, was it so bad to be born?" I felt a little lump on the side of the head and I kissed it and said, "Oh, that's what that squishy thing was!" The baby had had its head tilted to the side and I tore a little on the right side of my vagina because of that.

I moved the baby off my chest for a second to see what gender we had made together and I saw she was a very pretty girl. I Knew we had a girl through the whole last trimester of my pregnancy, I just knew. Ross had seen it was a girl right away, but he remembered I wanted to see for myself and not be told (Thank you for remembering, Ross!). I was examining her very long cord, which she had not only wrapped around her neck but also her body, it was really pretty shade of bluish purple. Wise baby, protecting herself from a cord prolapse like that.

I was amazed with how girly and delicate her hands and feet were, Gabriel's were so huge compared to hers! She was so girly from the start, very pretty, delicate and SO loud; she is woman, and we hear her ROAR! I decided to get back in the still warm and inviting birth tub to clean of just a bit, covered in blood and meconium as we were. We got out after Ross took the bloody sheets and plastic off the bed and we crawled in and wrapped in our favorite wool quilt and settled in to nursing while we waited for the placenta. The cord had turned white and limp, so we tied and cut it, I got up to push the placenta out in to a bowl, and it did not hurt like I was expecting it to. I looked it over and it was whole and intact and a bit heavier than I had expected. I smelled it for some reason, and it had a unique and kind of cool smell, nothing I would bottle, but interesting nonetheless. I ran a hot bath for myself so I could wash off a little better as I still had blood and meconium on my face. I talked to my mom and my dad on the phone, finally being honest and open with them about our birthing at home which was a relief. They were in awe, and not upset at all as far as I could tell. We settled into bed for the night until around 7:00 a.m., when Gabriel woke up to meet his sister. He came out and said, "Baby!! Meow, baby!!" I guess she sounds like a kitty. He gave her kisses and was so sweet; to this day he will never refuse to kiss 'his' baby, he will sometimes refuse to kiss Mama and Daddy, but never his baby.

After doing this I feel like I can do anything I put my heart in to, it is amazing to feel like that again. After my Cesarean Section with Gabriel, I did not feel like myself. A lot was taken away from me that day, not just the chance to push out a baby, but a lot of my 'self' was taken, a lot of my fire and spirit along with most of my confidence. I had been banking it all up since August 2006 when I had resolved to take control of my birthing, putting it all in layaway a little at a time, and I finally got it all back the night I had Violet, with interest! Ross says I even look different. I definitely feel different, I feel redeemed and proud of myself for accomplishing so much in such a short time. I also feel like I absolutely must help to spread this feeling to as many women as I can. I know that unassisted birth is not ideal for everyone, but for me, it is the only way I feel I could safely and securely give birth. For me, any interference at all, 'good' or 'bad', would have ruined my Violet's birth.

I respect the need for well-trained obstetricians in hospitals or operating rooms, in the cases when medical care is prudent. It isn't that I have something against doctors or hospitals, it is just, I personally do not need all that to give birth. I love and respect the work that midwives do, their wisdom and their dedication to a profession that is really unappreciated by our society at large. I have every intention on training as a midwife in the future when my children are a little older, not requiring my undivided attention and are no longer breastfeeding. So it is not as if I have something 'against' midwives, I simply would never have been comfortable being myself in front of a midwife, even if she was a friend, I would never have really been able to let go and just birth. I know that for sure. The simple truth is this: Ross is the only person who really knows what I am all about, he really knows what I need and want and he can do it without disturbing me or even without thinking, and in the moment of birthing, that is the most important thing, I think. We were the best midwives I could ask for. A great number of couples do not have the sort of relationship conductive to unassisted birth, and some do; a great number of women do not have a personality conductive to birthing alone, and again, some do. I had no real desire to be all-alone, I wanted Ross to be with me, idle but present, and that is what he was; it was perfect for us.

I think we in the birthing 'community' need to realize everyone has individual needs and desires, some need and desire to be completely alone, some want a midwife, some want their mothers, and some want an obstetrician and an epidural. And we all need to respect and support those needs and wants. All women need to have choices, many varied choices that they can choose from freely without worry of people thinking they are 'crazy' or 'weak' or 'radical'. I felt the need to keep our plans for an unassisted birth a secret among many of our family members and friends until after the fact because I could not deal with the fearful, rude and even downright snarky comments and 'looks' during my pregnancy if I were to be peaceful and happy. Which has since made me resolve as long as a woman has educated herself with accurate truthful information about all of her choices I have no place thinking (or saying) anything but supportive things, even if she has decided to have an elective Cesarean Section operation after being fully informed of risks and benefits.

I think we could all resolve to make sure women are well educated about their options for birth. It is in our hands, we have the ability to change things for the better, if only we would act to do so. We must let the well educated woman choose what is best for her and her family in birth, and then just let her choice be, whether or not we think it is the 'right' choice; it will make for happier, easier

pregnancies and a much more simple kind of birth.

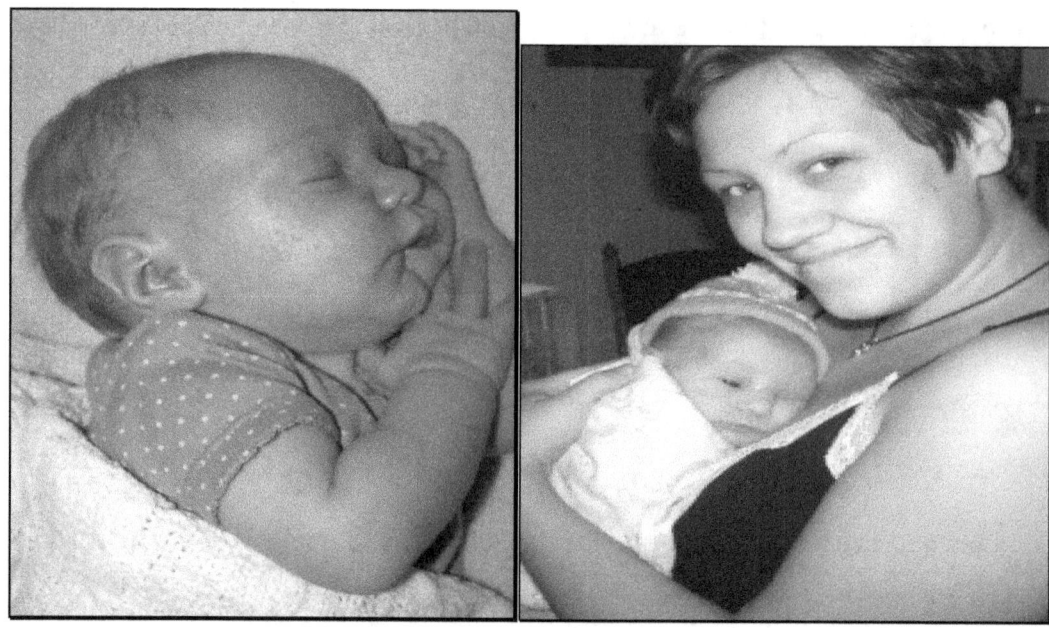

Mom	: Jasmine Rae Ojala
Dad	: Jonas Ross Ojala
City State	: Minneapolis, MN
Age at birth	: 22, 41weeks pregnant
Birth	: Second
Baby's Name	: Violet Hope
Baby's Height	: 21 1/4 inches
Baby's Weight	:10 lbs 3 oz

Morvryn Sage Leon Brown

At the 21st of September 2007 I woke up at around 7:00 a.m. and felt like I was getting my period. It felt like those cramps I always get right before the bleeding starts, but those "cramps" came every twenty minutes. I was confused, because I thought pressure waves would feel different, like they would start from the back and work their way to the front…. I decided to have a normal day. By about 4:00 p.m. those odd cramps were about twelve minutes apart. I thought it might be best to call the midwife, since I had planned a homebirth and I was alone at home. My husband is in the Army and he was in Alabama at the time in the field while I was at our house in Kentucky.

Ann, our midwife, came and said I was not opening yet, but I might want to get David, my husband, home, so he would not have to start driving home when I am already in labor. We were both worried he would drive like a nutcase. So at 4:30 p.m. we called Red Cross America and told them I would be in labor and we would need the Army to send David home. Then the midwife went back home thinking David would be on his way.

Well, those cramps continued they did not change they just came more often. At first I was surprised and tensed up and they were painful. But then I decided to stop listening to my head and let my body do the work. So really every time they came I went on my hands and knees and I shook my butt I was Hoola-Dancing the whole time.

When I was moving, the pain just changed into pressure. It was not bad anymore at all and I thought I managed really well. I kept on calling my husband to see if he was on his way because I started to realize that this was it. But he had not heard anything yet from Red Cross. He wanted me to call our midwife, but I felt good alone at home and did not want anybody else around. I started filling the pool though and I put on some candles and burned some sage to clear the atmosphere in the room. In between doing all this I had to go on my hands and knees and shake my hips all the time of course.

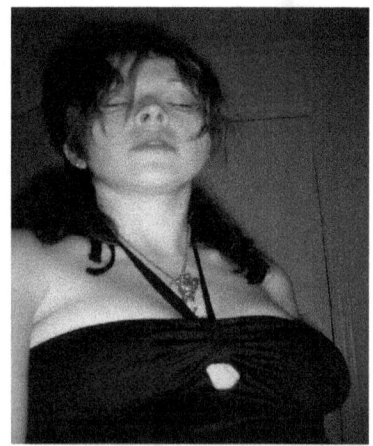

Well, I made the pool water too hot at first and then too cold and I ended up having to boil water on the stove, go down and hands on knees, bring the water to the pool, go down on hands and knees, go back to the kitchen and boil more water.

At about 10:15 p.m. I was ready to get into the water. The pressure waves came every five minutes. So I called my midwife. She came about twenty minutes later and told me I was already at 7 cm. I was surprised! At about 10:25 p.m. Red Cross Kentucky called me to let me know that they had just called Red Cross Alabama. I was mad! It took them from 4:30 p.m. to 10:25 p.m. to call from Kentucky to Alabama. Since my midwife usually works for the Amish here I told them I should have sent one of the Amish guys on the horse. They might have been faster. I figured if it took Red Cross Kentucky so long to get with Red Cross Alabama, it might take them a few hours to get with David's unit and I started to think that he might not make it.

Well, I went in the water and from then on everything went smooth. The water felt great and I kept on doing my little dance. We had only candlelight on and I listened to the "Rilke Projekt"… a cd with poetry. I had wanted an unassisted birth at first, so our midwife knew not to talk to me too much and just to let me do my thing. And she did. She started talking later, but since she talked in English, it did not bother me at all. I focused on the German words from the cd.

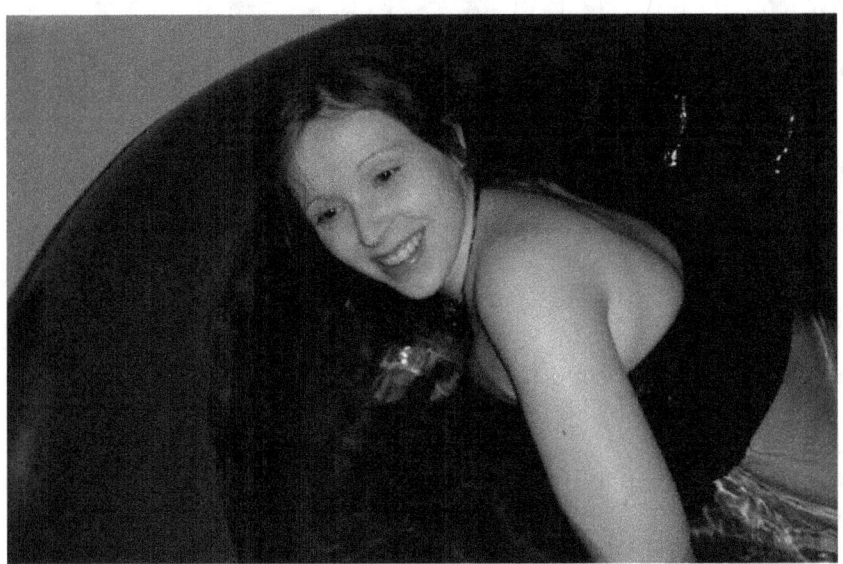

Ann was sitting next to the pool holding the phone close to me so I could talk to my husband. I sounded like a radio journalist who does the sport. "Okay honey, hold on. I won't be able to talk for a minute…. All right, I am fine. Do not worry, okay… It is not bad at all. It probably sounds worse than it is…"

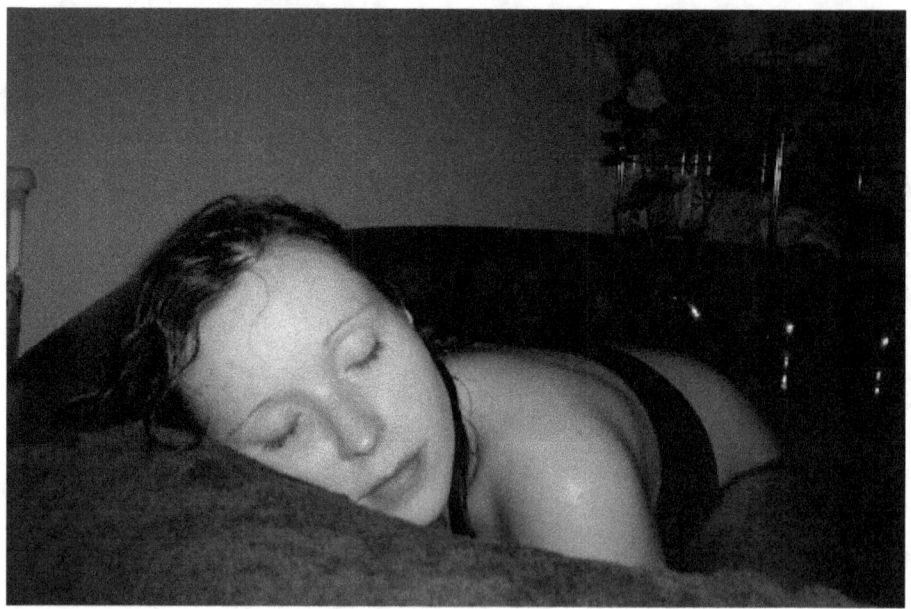

I do not know when I started to feel "pushy".... But I know that I got really tired. I had not slept more than about 3 hours the night before and I almost fell asleep in the pool once. When I started to feel pushy I wanted to have my ears underneath the water. I don't know why, but it felt great. I felt a lot of pressure in my hips and at one point it really hurt. I noticed that I had allowed my head to come back into the game. So I talked to my brother Sebastian. See, he died when he was 17 and I had chosen him to be my baby boy's guardian. While I was pregnant I dreamt about Sebastian a lot. So I talked to him and told him to help my son to dance right through my body. And it worked. I relaxed and I felt pressure and I felt exhausted, but no pain anymore.

I really believe that pain most of the time is caused by our thinking, our fear and our "tensing up".... That is why I hate it when people tell me I had an easy birth. Well yes, I prepared for it and worked for it. And I do not have a high pain tolerance at all. I just believe that I should do what is best for the baby and not what is easiest for me. So to me that meant NO DRUGS unless there is an emergency. It was clear to me that I had to put my baby first. That is why I practiced meditation and hypnosis during the pregnancy. Most people seem to think there are those who birth easily and those who have bad births. I think there are those who are scared and tense and have a bad birth because of that and those who are relaxed and feel safe and have a good birth... And of course there are a few who have problems and really need help during birth. But at least 97 – 98 % of all women could and should have good births. That does not mean it always has to be absolutely painless, but the pain will be so you are able to take it without going insane. And anyway, who ever said that pain always has to be bad? But that is me.

Well, I cannot tell you how long I had my head underneath the water. Finally I decided I needed to go pee. Ann told me I could pee in the pool, but I was not willing to do that. So I climbed out of the pool (hard work) and went to the bathroom. In the hallway the water broke. Then I decided to walk through the house to speed things up. Ann following behind me with the phone.... And then, right when I was at the house door I felt like I had to get back into the pool right away. So I tried to run... not a good idea... I put my hands inside myself to see where my baby was and he was close. I had my hands inside myself almost all the time. My midwife thankfully encouraged me to do that.

When I climbed back into the pool I started to make odd noises. I was worried that my husband on the phone might freak out about time. He was driving home at this time. I told him it did not hurt; it just helps to make this sound…. I could feel my baby's head on my fingers moving down. I kept on thinking about that one sentence I read in the HypnoBirthing book (which is all I used for preparation)… "Breathing love, nurturing life." I kept on saying that to myself as I breathed my baby down. And then I could see his hair. His head came out, got back in, came out… My legs started shaking and I had no control over them anymore. I was amazed by that and just starred at them. Ann and her assistant Elsie held my legs for me, because I was not able to change back to my hands and knees like I wanted to. From that moment on my body went numb. I had expected the ring of fire… but nothing. From that moment on I was not even exhausted anymore.

I think some endorphins kicked in. I felt only joy now and I watched my son's head coming out, then his shoulders, then the rest of his beautiful little body. A minute later he was on my chest looking at me like he was saying, "What happened? Where am I?" My husband on the phone said, "Is everything alright?"

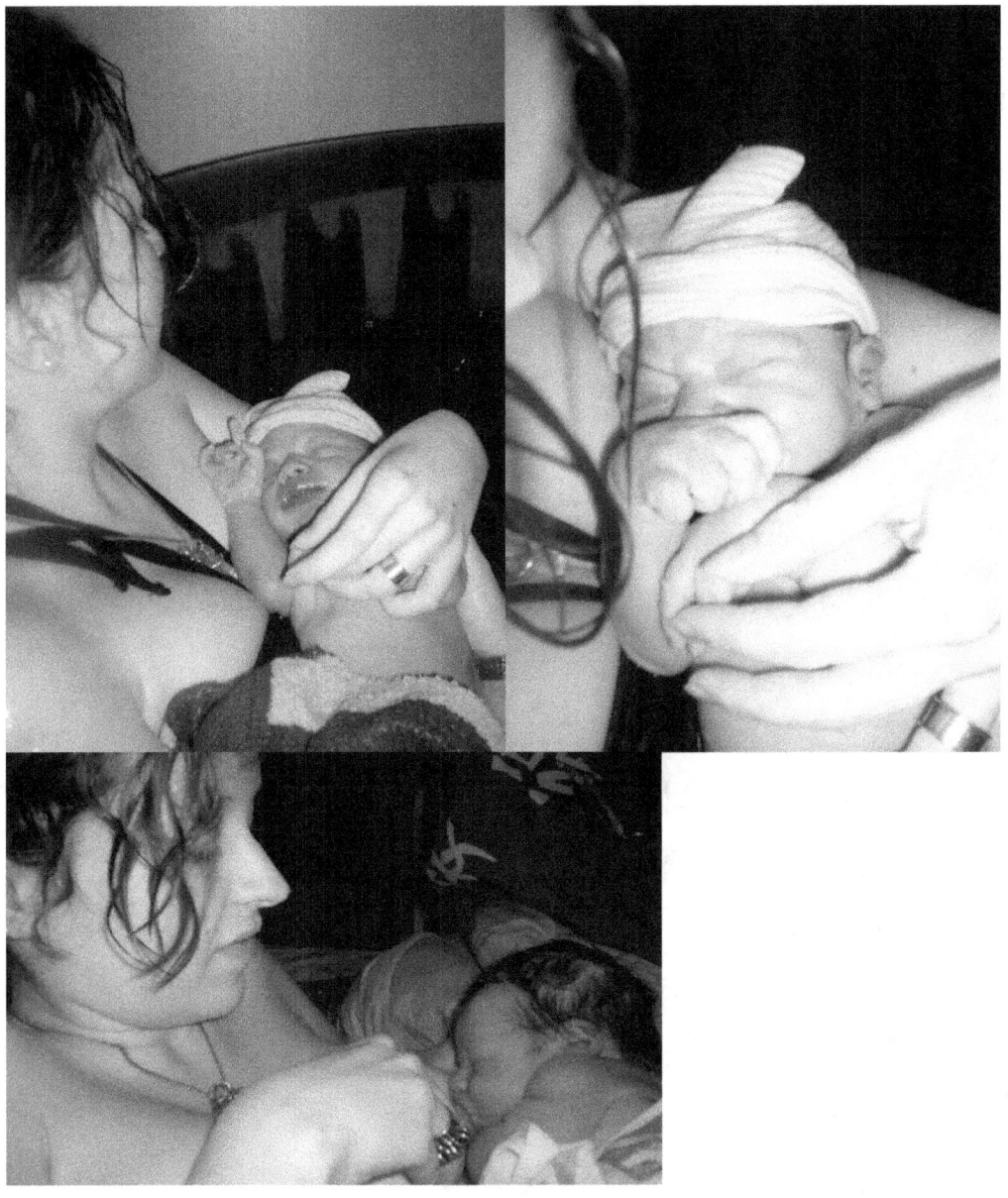

and our son turned his head to see where that voice had come from. Then Ann

checked him while he was still on me. He was fine, but he started crying. Nearly

broke my heart to hear that!

I nursed a bit and then we waited for the placenta. It did not take long, but to me it felt like it took forever. When the placenta was out Ann checked me and I went to take a shower. Then my husband came home and I went to bed with my two boys. Our son Morvryn was born at 1:15 a.m. Of course I could not sleep that night. So I called my family in Germany and at about 7:00 a.m. I got up and made breakfast.

Since then I have felt fine. I had no after pains and Morvryn is gaining weight fast. That was thirteen days ago and now the bleeding has almost stopped. I am back to my before pregnancy weight and my body feels like this miracle never happened. Sometimes I wake up at night and look at my boy next to me, just to make sure it was not just a dream. The only bad thing now is that Ann told me I

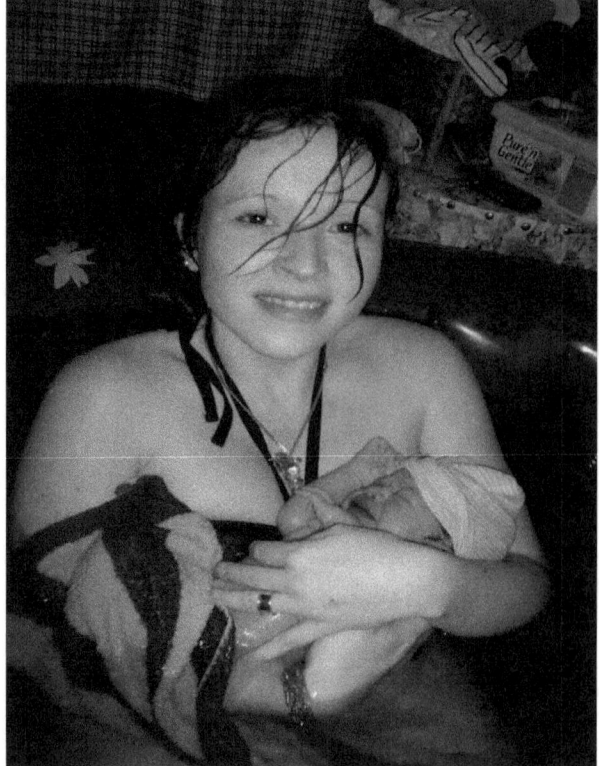 am not allowed to have sex for six weeks. All the best to all of you!

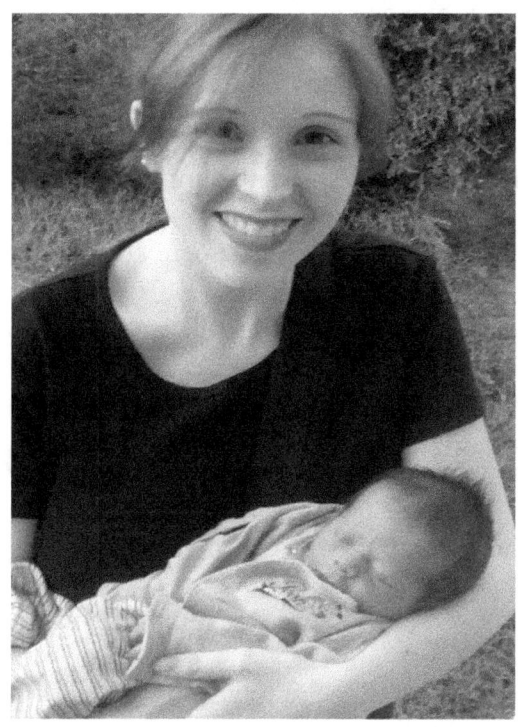

Mom	: Saskia Steidel-Brown
Dad	: David Scott Brown
City State	: Oak Grove, KY
Age at birth	: 25
Birth	: First
Baby's name	: Morvryn Sage Leon
Baby's Height	: 18 inches
Baby's Weight	: 3402 gram

Gianna Belle

I woke up Sunday, April 1st just feeling exhausted. All day long, there was nothing that I could do to gain my energy back, and so I spent most of the day in bed resting and sleeping. I couldn't remember the last time I had spent so much time sleeping! Closer towards the evening, I rolled out of bed for the second time and decided to make my way downstairs. Around this time, I noticed contractions again – and every now and then, I'd feel one in my back. By the time 9:00 p.m. arrived I was having regular contractions and feeling most everyone in my back first. However, they were totally manageable and I really didn't even think much of these contractions except for the back pain. When I spoke to a friend on the phone and told her what I was experiencing, she suggested calling the midwife. So I did, and at my midwife's recommendation, I went upstairs and checked myself. Whew! I was about 3cm dilated, and could literally feel the sack bulging out of my cervix. At that point I began to question if I would be having the baby soon! Ha! I told my midwife what I discovered and she asked if I thought that tonight would be my night. "I honestly have no idea. I mean, part of me thinks that surely something must be going to happen soon…." - - but I couldn't guarantee to her that I was in active labor at that point! She suggested us putting the boys to bed and then seeing if something happened after that. I don't know how she knows these things!

Immediately after putting the boys down for the night, I crawled into bed and laid on my side thinking about these contractions. It was seriously starting to irritate me that I couldn't tell which way things were going. I felt out of touch with my body. Thirty minutes passed, and Corey spoke with the midwife, asking her to come on out. Since she lives an hour and 15 minutes away, we knew it would take her a little bit to get here but it was also just after 10:00 p.m. at that point, so the roads were more than likely clear for her to get here a bit sooner than normal. I was still second guessing everything – and telling myself that we were probably having her out here for nothing. I honestly thought at that point that we'd just be sending her back home with no baby in our arms yet. Corey said, "Better safe than sorry, though. Let's just see what happens."

Corey pulled out some chux pads and ran a hot bath for me. I got in there and little did I know that it would be a few hours before I climbed out. The hot water helped me relax and made the back contractions ease up quite a bit. Thank goodness! While I was in the tub, though, the contractions gradually picked up and between 11:30 p.m. and 1:00 a.m., I was in full blown labor. With each and every single contraction I motioned to Corey and he put his hand on my lower back just right to put pressure on my spine and ease the pain. It helped a lot. I absolutely needed him there doing that for me and he was just awesome.

The contractions grew intense, and I could feel the powerful waves start to push baby down and slowly start to spread my hip bones apart. The baby was moving down further and further, and pretty soon, I could feel such a pressure on my butt and the baby's head at the opening. Now I was softly moaning and involuntarily pushing with each contraction. "That's good! That's what we want!" my midwife spoke gently. She grabbed her Doppler and kept a check on baby's heartbeat here and there. "Baby sounds good! Everything is going great! You are doing PERFECT!" she said. I could really start to feel baby's head coming out, and for some reason I started to arch my back in the water. "If you're going to have this baby in the water, then you'll have to keep your butt below the water. If not, then let's get out and try something different" my midwife told me. I felt like I was trying but to no avail to get the baby down past a certain point, so my midwife directed me to come forward and get up on my feet (with help, of course!). Corey and the midwife assistant helped me up, and before I knew it I was standing up in the tub and really pushing the baby out. Her head had crowned and more was coming out when the midwife directed the birth team to help me out of the tub and let me squat on the floor beside it.

Squatting, how could I have forgotten about squatting? It works So well and feels SO good birthing a baby that way. I should have been in that position all along. They helped me squat on the floor and the baby's head popped out so fast after that…and then the shoulders and everything else came out in practically one big motion. WHOOSH! It felt great! The baby was covered in the creamy vernex and I reached down to pick up my child "Oh my baby! Oh my baby!! I can't believe it!"…after a few seconds it actually occurred to me to see who I had just birthed, so I quickly looked down there and proudly, loudly exclaimed,

"…and it's a GIRL! Oh my goodness! A girl!! Her name is Gianna Belle! She's

so beautiful! A girl, Corey, a GIRL!!" I held her so close, and kissed her and

loved her. She was just sucking all over her hands and was totally ready to nurse

right from the get-go! I couldn't believe that either! This was a first for me! It

was a bit before I could nurse her though, and she pitched a fit over it too!

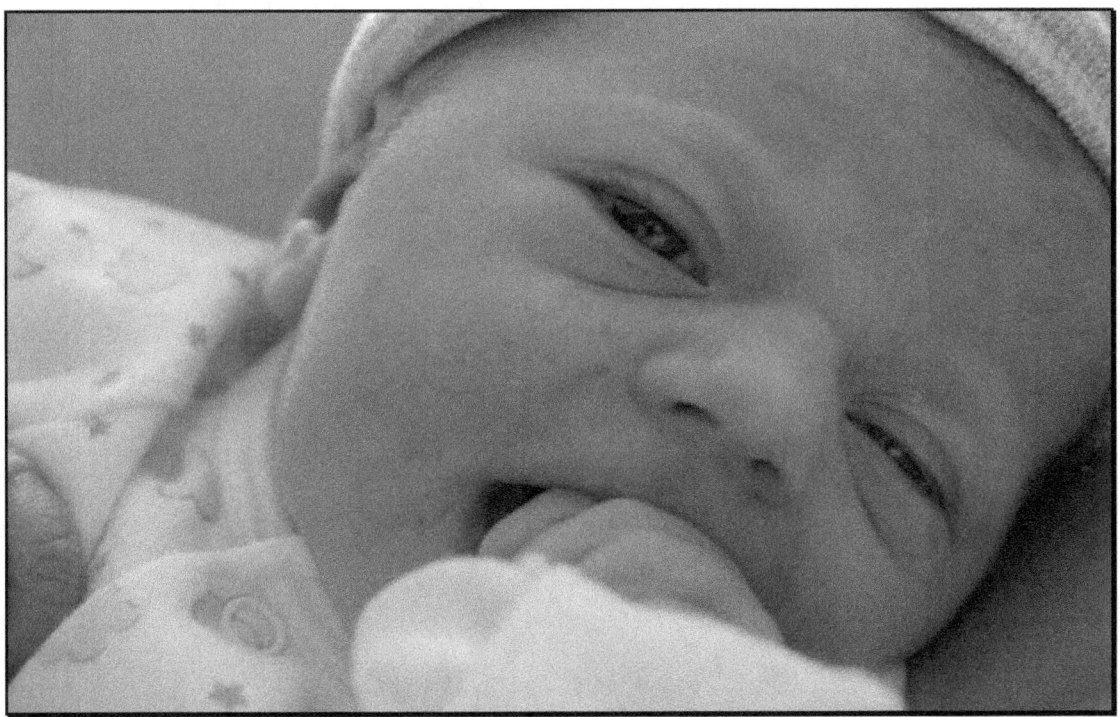

The birth team let the water out of the tub, cleaned it and ran a new, sparkly

hot bath for me and Gianna. Within minutes, we were back in the tub relaxing

and bonding. My midwife was also waiting for the cord to stop pulsating so that

we could cut it. She kept checking it every so often, but it was a good 35 minutes before it stopped pulsating, and she set it up so Corey could come over and cut the cord. Then we had to wait on the placenta. Corey held Gianna now while I got in a in a squatting position in the tub to push out the placenta. After that, my birth team cleaned me off in the tub, and then helped me to my bed. Corey brought over Gianna, and I put her up to me to nurse, which she was past ready to do. She latched on like a champ and had such a strong suck! Whew! That kicked my uterus in gear again with those intense contractions! After that, my midwife gave Gianna a thorough checkup and found that she was very tiny indeed – weighing in at only 6 lbs 9 oz and 19 inches long. Everything about her is perfect. God has blessed us with another healthy baby!

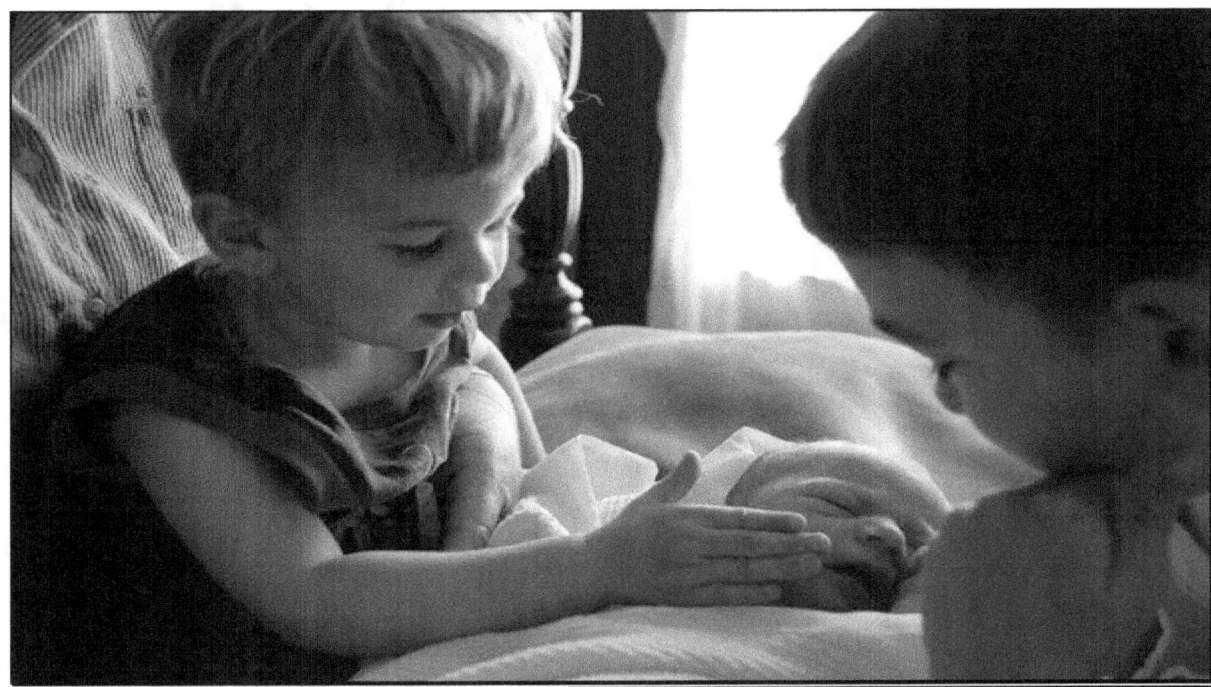

Mom   :Amber
Baby's Name :Gianna Belle
Birth   :Third
Baby's Weight:6 lbs. 9 oz.
Baby's Height :19 in. long
Born at 1:12 AM, April 2, 2007

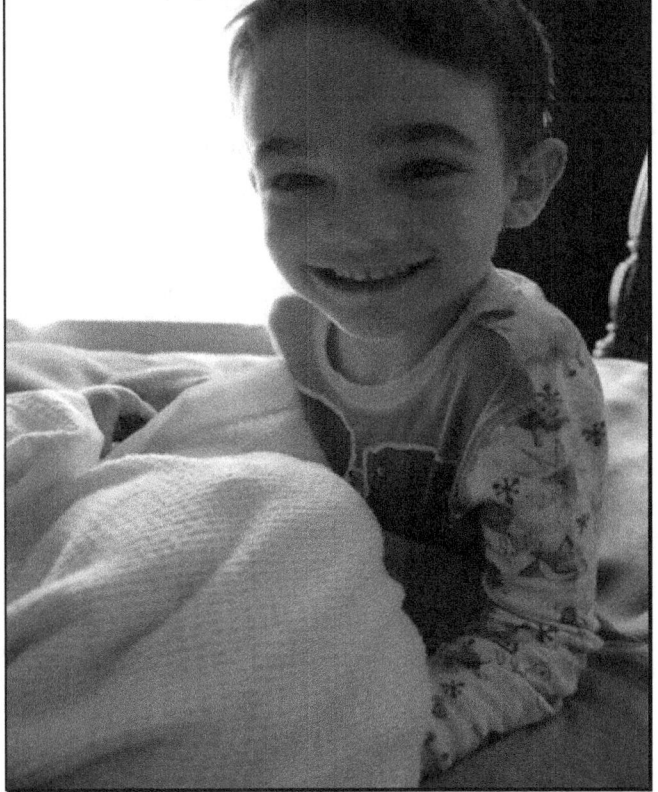

Anayi and Eliyah

Blood. My heart froze that night in the bathroom. Everything vanished in my focus except the blood. Fourteen weeks pregnant, out of the danger zone I had thought, yet all I could see was blood. I yelled for my roommate who helped me to my bed. I lay there trembling in shock, sobbing. Having been stunned by a surprise pregnancy during a particularly difficult time in my life, I had come not only to accept but also cherish this little life growing within me. I was going to be a mother again! But fears icy grip paralyzed me that night. Was I going to lose this life so soon?

The ER visit was routine; long waits, a hard bed in a cool room and a doctor's exam. They found nothing wrong. I waited a while longer for a quick ultrasound to make sure everything was ok. By 3:00 a.m. I was physically exhausted, bleary eyed from the events of the evening and emotionally spent. As the machines warmed up, my heart was tensed with fear. What if something was wrong? What if the heartbeat that I had heard a week before was no longer there? My mind rushed as the technician began her exam.

The look on her face confirmed my fears. I could see it in her eyes, intently looking with a frown at the screen, and then at my belly as she searched it with her machine. My heart sank as she returned her focus to me and stated coolly, "You haven't had an ultrasound yet have you? Her words pregnant with some dreaded knowledge. "No, I anxiously replied, wanting to scream but staying in surreal control, "Why, what's wrong?" She kept looking at her screen, moving the wand over my small but growing belly. The icy dread pounded in my heart, amplifying as every second passed. She finally responded quietly, "Because there are two."

Two?! My heart flipped as a flood of profound relief rushed over me; my baby was ok! Yet in the same instant my mind seemed to explode as it struggled to comprehend the word *two*. Overcome with so many conflicting emotions, all I could do was laugh hysterically and cry at the same time. "Oh my god, you aren't freaking serious." I exclaimed in utter disbelief, "You can't be serious, there are two???" She turned the screen towards me as if to prove her point. I could see their two little heads, and two beating hearts. I was having twins. Initial shock wore off to the busyness of making plans. Pregnancy, already such an amazing milestone in a woman's life, the carrying of my twins became something sacred. I craved the beauty of precious memories like the ones that I treasured with my first daughter.

My first birth, though in a hospital had been natural and without drugs, an amazing and empowering experience. I was hoping for a similar experience again. Little did I know that everything was to be more complicated with twins. I quickly realized that in most clinics, certified nurse midwives (CNMs) would not take twin cases. They are considered too high risk. I wasn't thrilled with my choices, but nevertheless started seeing an obstetrician. I was even less thrilled as I began to understand the hospital policies regarding twin births.

As my pregnancy progressed, I grew more dissatisfied with my lack of options. My chances of a C- Section were high, and there was the possibility that I could deliver one baby naturally, and the second by section. I couldn't imagine trying to take care of two infants and recover from major surgery at the same time. I was still determined to birth my babies as naturally as possible. I strongly felt that interventions like drugs would lead to more interventions and a higher risk of complications. I also wanted to experience the profound and exhilarating experience of an unmedicated birth. Burned in my memory was the feeling of that last painful push and then the sudden relief of emptiness and painless elation as my daughter was born and she gazed for the first time at me with those large blue eyes.

At 26 weeks, I hit a small complication. There was still plenty of time, but my second baby was presenting breech. My obstetrician knew I wanted a completely unmedicated labor, but the hospital policy was that every mother of twins has an epidural. She graphically described to me what a breech delivery would look like and why the epidural would be necessary: the doctor would reach her hand into my contracting uterus and pull the baby down and out of my birth canal by her feet. This was called a *breech extraction*, and from what I could ascertain, the only way they would deliver a breech baby vaginally.

I was not thrilled, to say the least. Appalled would be a better description. I had read about breech deliveries and knew they were highly uncommon in the hospital, but was this entirely necessary? Traumatic memories of a manual extraction of my placenta with my first daughter, a similar and excruciating procedure, left me crystal clear on what I did and *did not* want inside my uterus. I was not about to allow someone's hand go back up into that very private place. My uterus was for my babies only, and they were coming OUT, I wanted nothing else going IN there!

As the fearful scenarios were unfolded to me, and reality told me that I was most likely in for a traumatizing experience, the excitement and anticipation of my upcoming birth gave way to fear and doubt. Frustrated and hoping that there were other options, I began looking into the alternatives of birthing centers and direct-entry midwives.

I was familiar with the idea of home-birth from friends and acquaintances that had done it. And though I didn't fit into the all-natural, home-birth stereotype, I was never the type to be content with the mainstream either. I enjoyed thinking outside of the confines of my box in many areas of my life, and although this was a bit outside that box for me, I was cautiously open to the idea. I decided that there could be no harm in exploring the possibility. Though many did not take twin cases, I was quickly referred to Marilyn Milestone, a direct-entry midwife who had 25 years of experience, who had delivered several sets of home-birth twins.

The way she managed twins was that I would see a perinatologist at the university hospital who would send her all the lab reports and ultrasound findings, and we would take things step by step. If we were all comfortable with the way things were by the end of the pregnancy, I could proceed with a home-birth. If not, I would give birth in the hospital. The freedom of choice felt like a breath of fresh air after feeling so confined by hospital policies and practices. I decided to transfer my care to this perinatologist so at least I would have the option in the end.

My pregnancy entered the last stretch as I began my 30th week. My breech baby had turned vertex, a very good sign. And they were both growing concordantly. With each baby having her own placenta and sac, I was in the lowest risk category for twins. But though things were going well, I was still not sure if I was going with the midwives or not. I still had a major issue with my insurance company paying, even though the cost would be minimal compared to the astronomical costs of a medicated hospital birth. My delivery date was drawing nearer, and I still had not established care with my midwives due to this small but important glitch, though we kept in touch from time to time.

I was 34 weeks along when my doctor discovered that I was 4 1/2cm dilated. I had felt nothing other than constant Braxton-hicks contractions, but nothing to alert me that I was in labor. I went on immediate bed rest, knowing that a delivery at this stage would definitely be in the hospital, and I would probably have very small, preemie NICU babies. Whatever I decided to do, I knew I wanted those babies to be healthy and strong, so keeping them inside as long as possible was my sole focus.

But the days slowly turned into weeks and my babies soaked up every extra ounce of nourishment my body provided them. Time seemed to stand still. By 36 weeks I went off my bed rest and still nothing happened. Large and very uncomfortable, I began to think that I was never going to have these babies. That week I went in for my appointment, and another doctor checked me. By his measurement I was 5 cm dilated, and my contractions were regular, but not painful. I tried to tell him that I was not in labor, but he insisted I go over to labor and delivery to make sure.

I knew the procedure well, having gone in for some false alarms; they don't allow you to eat until they are convinced you are not in labor. That can take anywhere from two to ten hours. And that long without food for a ravenous mother of twins is an eternity! Annoyed but afraid to go against his authority, I grudgingly went over, but not before the rebel in me wandered around the hospital for a while and ate a big lunch.

When they determined what I already knew, I was indeed *not* in labor; they still decided I should stay at the hospital. The doctor on duty was concerned with the slim chance of a uterine infection, being that I was so far dilated and 90 effaced. Another fear was that my labor would be quick and I would not make it to the hospital in time. My labor with my firstborn had been 4 ½ hours from beginning to end. I lived 35 minutes away from the hospital when the roads were clear; congested, more like an hour. I understood their concern, though in the back of my mind I wondered if they were attempting to control the situation. It was written all over my charts that I was planning on having a home-birth, and the overwhelming consensus in the hospital was that I was crazy to even think of such a preposterous idea.

What they didn't know when I entered the labor and delivery floor that week was that I had all but given up on the home-birth. After being given the run-around, I finally realized that there was no way my insurance would cover the midwives, and I had no extra money to pay them. Still being so many weeks before my due date and the doctors predicting delivery any minute, I had pretty much resigned myself to the fact that I was going to have these babies before I left the hospital. My last hope was to fight for the kind of labor experience I wanted in the hospital and hope that I got a doctor who was understanding enough to allow it.

So the hospital became my new home. Rayyan, my four-year-old crammed in my hospital bed with me at night. My sister, who came to live with me for a time to help, slept on the little couch they provided. The babies' daddy came to visit.

And still we waited and waited. All bets were off at that point, I had far surpassed everyone's expectations.

Not having much else to do, and wanting to prepare myself for my natural hospital labor, I had my sister bring me some books to re-read. I devoured *The Thinking Woman's Guide to a Better Birth* by Henci Goer in one sitting, scribbling down the questions that had been burning in my mind. Could I decline the epidural? Could I use positions that were most comfortable or would I have to labor and deliver on my back (an excruciatingly uncomfortable position already)? Could I hold my babies immediately after they were born or would they be taken from me? Would I have to be induced immediately after the first baby was born? If the second turned breech, could I try to deliver without the extraction as long as she wasn't in distress?

The longer I stayed, the more questions I had about what my birth would look like, and the more I disliked the answers. One late night after about a week in the hospital, I sneaked down to the labor floor and asked a nurse if she'd let me take a peek at the room that I would deliver in, the ominous Operating Room. Looking in, I envisioned with vivid clarity the frustrating picture the doctors had painted for me. There I was, lying flat on my back on that hard little table in the middle of a bright, sterile room. My feet in stirrups no less! Epidural in place (though with the option not to use the drug unless necessary) and strapped to various machines beeping around me. Bright lights glaring down on me, and a myriad of strangers (perinatologist, nurses, residents, anesthesiologist, and pediatricians, about ten people in all) packed into this small little room ready to take my babies the moment they were born. All watching with curious interest this strange and primitive woman who wanted to have her twins without drugs. At that moment my hopes of having a gentle and memorable birth shattered into pieces. And then a surge of angry defiance welled up within me. The timid rebel, until now too intimidated by the system, suddenly emerged with sheer determination and resolve. That would *not* be me in there!

With unwavering clarity, I called my midwife the next morning. I told her I didn't care what it took, I had made it to 37 weeks and I was going straight home to have my babies there, in the comfort of my own home, with the people who loved and supported me surrounding me. And that's exactly what I did.

Eight days into my hospital stay the doctors gave me the option to induce or go home. I didn't think twice. Strangely triumphant, feeling that I had won some unseen war of wills, I packed my belongings and was never so happy to be going home. Not knowing how much time I had, I quickly rushed to get the supplies needed for my home birth. The anticipation and excitement I felt was invigorating. My babies were big and healthy. They were both vertex. I felt a profound sense of relief knowing I was not going to have to fight my whole way through my labor. In the competent hands of women who trusted the natural birthing process, all I would have to do was relax and let my body do its job.

Friday morning comes: 3/4/05. I am 38 weeks and 1 day. Everyone, including the doctor (who wants to induce at this point) thinks it's time these babies came. Rayyan wakes me up at 7:30 in the morning and exclaims excitedly, "c'mon mom, were gonna get these babies coming' today!" So I drink some red raspberry leaf tea, and we waddle around my apartment complex as fast as a full-term woman with twins possibly can. We were quite a sight.

When I noticed a dribble of liquid run down my leg later that day, I was ecstatic. I stared at the father of my babies, and exclaimed, "I think that's my water! I gotta call everyone!" Filled with excitement and anticipation that my long awaited day had finally come, I called my mother, sister, best friend and midwives with my news. These babies were indeed coming today.

By the time everyone arrived, my labor was well underway. I was resting comfortably on my couch surrounded by my favorite pillows, breathing through my contractions, eating a bit here and there to keep my strength up. The labor grew intense, but in between contractions I was joking around about what the neighbors must be thinking or text messaging updates to my friends (who did not know I was laboring at home until after it was over). It was so comforting to have my family around me, experiencing this amazing event with me. And at every turn, I reminded myself what I would have had to be doing if I had been in the hospital. Through a particularly difficult contraction I wincingly moaned to my midwives, "Right about now is when I'd be taking the drugs! You sure you don't have any in your bags?"

It took an hour and a half after my bag of waters completely ruptured for Anayi to make her entrance. As her head crowned I vividly remember as one of the midwives held my gaze, my whole being focused on her intense blue eyes while she coached me to breathe in short bursts as the baby's head emerged. My whole body bore down to urge her gently into the world, and that moment of physical relief and emotional elation flooded over me as she was born. The sudden absence of pain and utter tranquility of my body in contrast to the intense contractions I had just experienced was indescribable. 5 lbs 12 oz, looking just like her daddy; Anayi was born into my arms, on my living room floor.

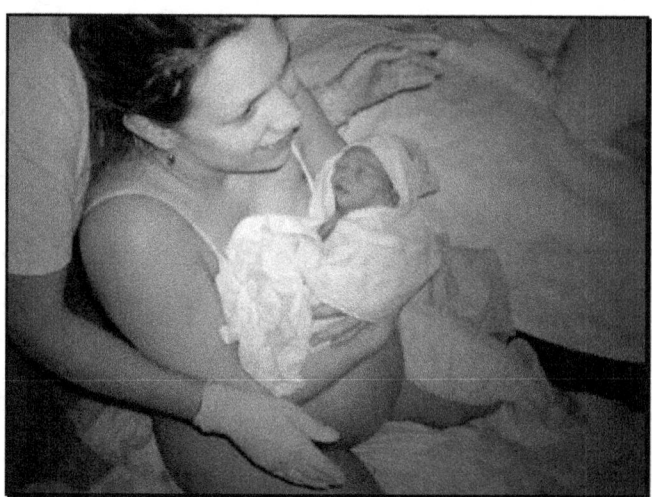

Following her birth, I had an hour of complete rest, where my body did nothing; a sort of calm in the center of the storm. I was no longer in labor. The midwives monitored Baby B, who was doing fine, enjoying her only time she would have my womb to herself. Anayi and I had time to bond and breast-feed and relax before I started feeling contractions again, and even then, they were spaced well apart and not incredibly intense.

Had I been in the hospital, I would not have enjoyed this peaceful time. The doctors made it clear that within minutes of the first birth, they would do everything in their ability to get my labor going again. And if after rupturing my membranes and administering pitocin, my body had still refused to work within their time frame, I could have faced a section. How grateful I was to be at home!

The midwives were comfortable allowing me to labor when I was ready, for which I was very thankful. With the pain and intensity still vividly fresh in my mind, I was *not* ready to push out another baby anytime soon! If there was one thing I felt from the midwives, it was their overwhelming confidence in the birthing process, and the absence of fear and worse case scenarios. They were so reassuring. Their relaxed manner even calmed my mother, the biggest worrywart I know. What a difference it was from the fear-charged atmosphere of the hospital. And so I took my time. So long in fact, that we were getting close to having twins with separate birthdays!

About 5 ½ hours later, I was mentally ready to do it again. My second bag of waters broke and within ten minutes I felt the intense contractions and urge to push. Half jokingly I lamented that it wasn't fair to have to do this twice in one day! As her head pushed through the ring of fire, I remember frantically searching again for those blue eyes to focus on to make it through the final stretch. After twenty-five minutes of intensity, on my hands and knees, my preferred birthing position, Eliyah was born at 11:45 that night, 6 pounds, 2 ounces.

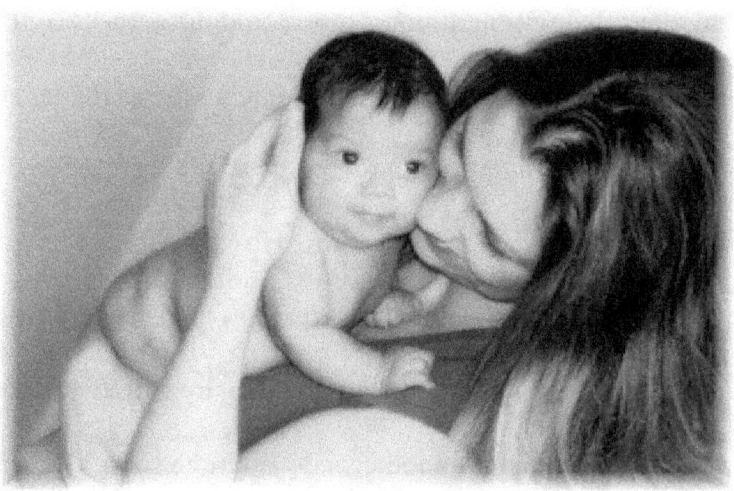

And so my precious girls were born, in the soft light of my living room, with a warm spring breeze floating through my open windows. Without the bright lights or sterile machinery beeping around me; born not into the hands of a waiting band of doctors ready to whisk them away, but into the arms of their loving mother.

People will say that it doesn't matter how your babies are born, as long as they are healthy. But the indescribable beauty of my birth and bonding I experienced with everyone present that day will last a lifetime. And the knowledge that I found the inner strength to birth my babies is empowering, and very helpful, because *now* is when the real work begins.

Kaden Reece

It was early April and I was pregnant with my second child. I was happy that he would be coming soon. I had lots of pre labor expansions on Thursday. It seemed I had a constant expansion all day that would get even tighter every five minutes. I had a midwife appointment and she asked if they were coming often, when she had felt how hard my belly was. I went to the chiropractor and was put into alignment, which felt great. My body was tingling and vibrating and I felt wonderful.

I went to Wal-Mart and locked my keys in the trunk of my car and my expansions had been getting closer together. They started coming every two minutes. My aunt came and got me and 3 hours after they were still at two minutes apart. Everyone wanted me to call the midwife I told her not to rush, as I wasn't in any discomfort at all. She came by and checked me I was 1-2 and 70% effaced so she left all her equipment and told me to call her when things started happening. I decided to get some sleep, as it didn't seem like they were dilating

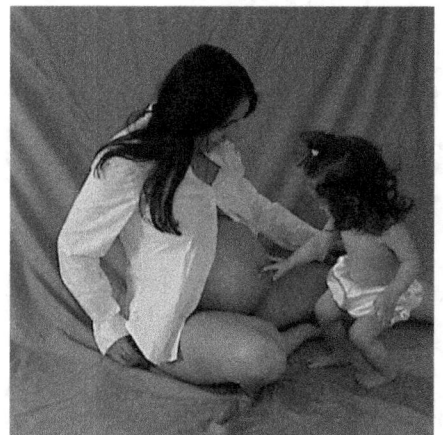

me any.

I woke up in the morning and they had stopped. I decided we would all go to the mall and walk around. I bought some raspberry leaf pills from the health store. The contractions were coming but it didn't feel like labor so we went to get some spicy food. We got it to go and when we got home found out they didn't season the wings. So I ate a couple jalapeno peppers had a teaspoon of castor oil in a milkshake made some loving and took a nap.

I woke up at 5:00 p.m. and I was having good expansions. They were

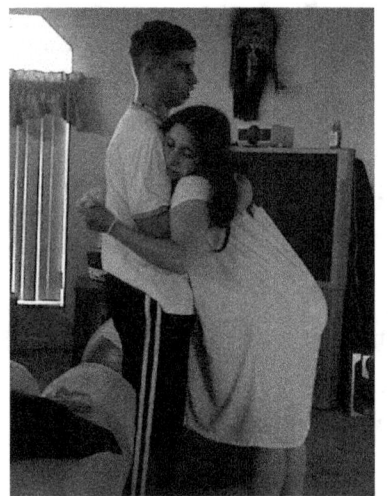

immediately something I had to pay attention to. They were one to two minutes apart so my husband called the midwife. I held on to my husband through many expansions and we would sway together and I walked in between them, which wasn't much time.

Then I began to feel tired from that and started using the birth ball and would walk in between. My mom and niece Alexis gave me reiki on my back and my husband stayed at my ear and said encouraging things. I kept saying I was a lioness because of this drawing by Pam England I had seen and loved of a woman giving birth with a lion head, which would make everyone laugh. (www.Birthingfromwithin.com)

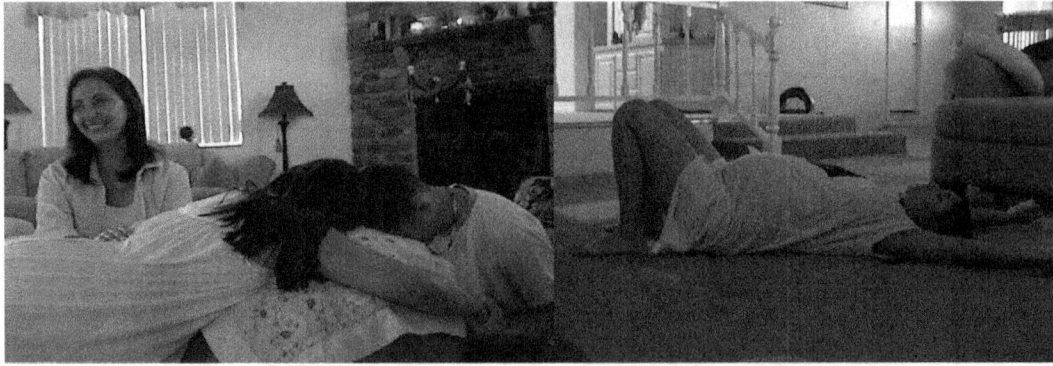

The midwife came and she checked me around 6:30 p.m. and said I was 3 cm dilated. So she encouraged me to try being upright more. So I walked and rocked on my husband and everyone sat in the living room and would give me drinks and sometimes I would go back on the birth ball if it were a tough one. I was so happy that I had a feeling the rushes were coming. I could feel it like a straight line very low in my belly and then it would build up and slow down. (That isn't how my last labor went.) So I had time to get into position, which was great. I had to be in position before the expansion peaked. At one point I had my sister count through the wave, so I would know that it was almost over.

My one-year-old daughter Jeweliana was so funny she kept making me laugh. She would come over to me and rub my hair, it was so sweet. Once she sat down at my butt and we all laughed that the baby was out and was walking already. She would poke my nose or dance a silly dance, which always made me smile.

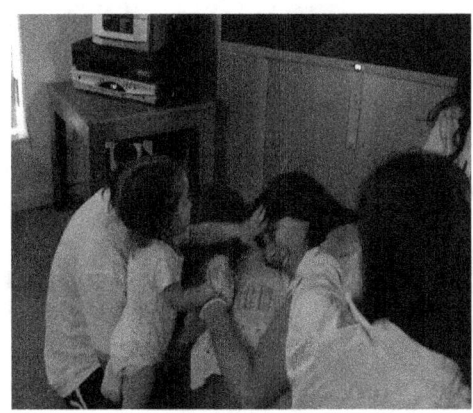

I took a shower with my husband Greg and we held onto each other and I loved how the water felt running down my body. Then I went back into the living room, I wanted to save the shower for later. The rushes were getting stronger and I was feeling like I wanted it to be over soon or for my water to break. I knew as soon as my water broke my son would be born.

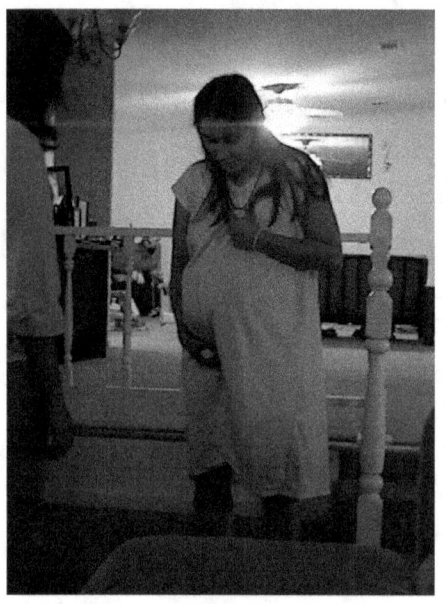

So I walked to my bedroom and took off my nightgown and the midwife checked me and said I was 7-8 cm and my bag was bulging. I lay on the bed and she helped me through a few expansions by saying, "let it be there" and I did and it felt great. Just like when I was in the living room and I would go inside the rush deep down and just be in that one spot on my body it felt so good. After each expansion I got this huge rush of oxytocin, which made me feel elated and in love. If I didn't focus on where the expansions were which was very low and strong then I felt like it was too tough to do. I would do great with five or so and then on the next one say I just want my water to break or I would say out loud "I can do this, feel it, breathe etc.". I had a list of encouraging things I wanted people to say to me and they did. My aunt had showed up and joined everyone in the living room.

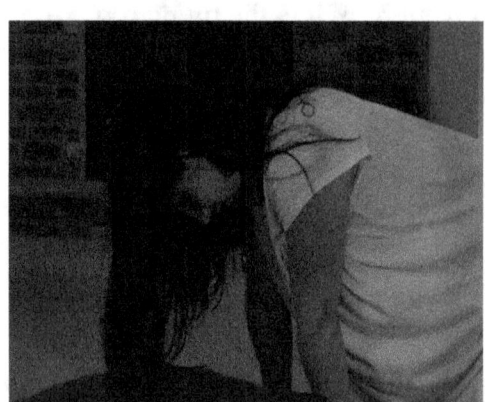

I went back into my bedroom as I felt it was getting close and then I called for my mom to come and she did. Then the other girls came and sat on the floor in my room quietly. I didn't want anyone to touch me and I danced and walked around my room the candles were lit and it was calm and peaceful.

I was starting to get bored in-between contractions, which was probably for about 30 seconds at this point and was wondering how much longer it was going to be. It was less than twenty minutes away! I didn't want all the people in there yet but there wasn't much time in between to tell them. I feel I handle labor much better alone so after I had some bloody show I decided to go get into the shower.

My husband sat on the sink and shut off the light so it was only candlelight. He sat quietly while I danced in the shower to a song that had started playing in my head…Every time we touch I get this feeling and every time we kiss I swear I can fly can't you feel my heart beat fast I want this to last I need you by my side… I haven't heard that song much and I didn't even know who sang it. But it has a great beat and I felt so great I was so happy and felt so connected to my baby it was beautiful. I was having so much fun it was so much better than being watched. I also got inspiration from my shampoo bottle, which said 10x stronger,

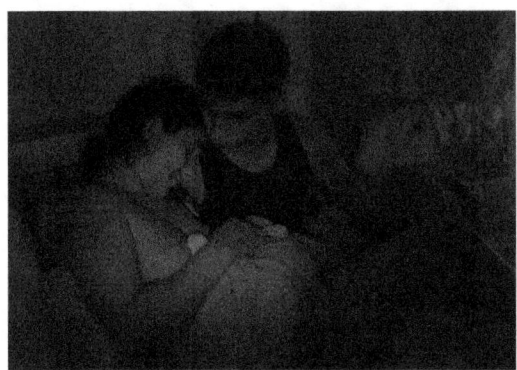

and my apricot facial scrub, which said, invigorating! I loved the rushes where I just felt them and let them do their thing; instead of resisting them, they were so much easier and very enjoyable. I could feel the oxytocin release in my body and rush through me it was amazing. I was having so much fun in that shower. My midwife opened the door and asked Greg something and I said "Shut the hell up!" My flow did not want to be interrupted. The next contraction was painful. Then Greg went to use the other bathroom and I went back into my trance, dancing around in the shower swaying to my son's birth dance with me.

My water broke with a huge gush it was so cool and loud! I yelled, "My water broke!!" with great excitement. Everyone had heard it too. My midwife Melissa came in and said "Okay you might want to get out now because the next contractions are going to be stronger." And as soon as she finished that sentence I had one and boy was it strong. I am surprised my daughter Jeweliana didn't wake up from when I banged on the shower wall. They tried to dry me off and took my shower cap off before the next one and I barely made it to my bed, which wasn't far. So I was on all fours on my bed until it was over and then I got on my back and felt the baby starting to come out. It was so cool I didn't feel that with my daughter's birth. I felt my body squeeze him so tight and push him down. I didn't even have to push. I felt his head starting to crown and the midwife gave me a hot compress and I held it against his bulging head. Greg sat down between my legs. The midwife and my mom and the nurse were on my right and my sister aunt and niece crowded at the bottom behind Greg. I said it burns he's coming out too fast I'm going to tear. The midwife said no you're not going to tear it's stretching great just blow. So I felt him moving down more and I still felt like I wasn't stretching enough so I quickly focused on opening up more by keeping an image of a lotus flower in my mind. Then I pushed and his head came out and I was holding his head and it felt so good I felt his face and rubbed his head gently. I said "I love you my baby, I love you." and I was waiting for the next expansion to push him out but it didn't come so the midwife said give a little push so I did and I pulled him up onto my chest. I did it all and I will never forget that moment or the amazement I felt.

He was so beautiful and peaceful. I just looked at him and told him I loved him so much and then I tried to nurse him, which he wasn't interested in for a while. He did such a great job and I put his little bear hat on his head and wrapped him in a blanket. He was wide eyed and I kept him nuzzled close to my chest. I kept feeling the cord and felt it pulsing blood into my little man. Everyone left the room and Greg watched as I held him and we got to know our son. Then the midwife came back to see about the placenta which came right out and then I cut his cord and Greg held him. After I cut the cord Melissa said "And now one are two."

I had a side wall tear and got three stitches. We did his newborn exam and he did the baby crawl and rolled over he got a ten on his Apgar and he weighed in at 5 lbs 12 oz and 19 inches long. My daughter Jeweliana came in a few hours later to meet him. She said so sweetly "babies" and gave him a kiss. We all fell asleep around 3:30 a.m. together. I am so happy it was in my home I wouldn't have in any other way. It was so perfect and I loved every minute of it. I am so grateful that he is so healthy and he is such a happy peaceful little man.

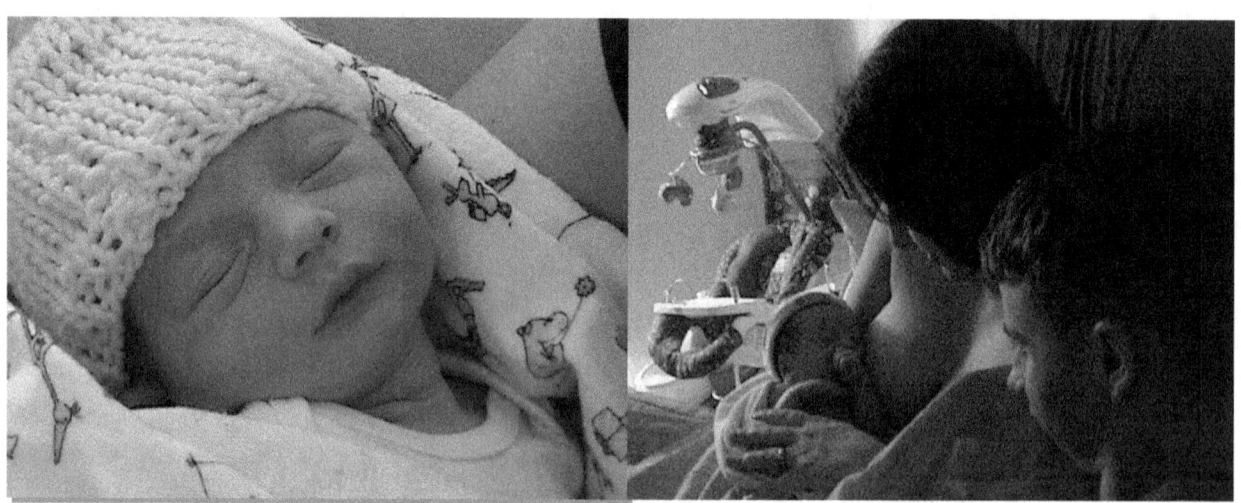

Mommy	:Jessica Levesque
Daddy	:Greg Levesque
City State	:Lakeland Fl
Age at birth	:23
Birth	:2
Baby's Name	:Kaden Reece
Baby's Height	:19 inches
Baby's Weight	:5lbs 10oz

About the Author

Jessica L. Levesque lives in Florida with her husband Greg and two children. She was born in New Jersey and raised in South-Eastern Massachusetts. She is a childbirth advocate, childbirth doula, Reiki Master/Teacher and stay at home mother. Her passion is to assist mothers in creating empowering and loving childbirth experiences. She hopes to restore positive uplifting views of childbirth. She intends to empower and inspire women to create the birth experiences they desire by helping them realize their inner strength. Her daughter Jeweliana was born naturally in a hospital birth center in 2005. Jessica's son Kaden was born at home in 2006. She encourages you to live an inspiring life filled with trust and beauty.

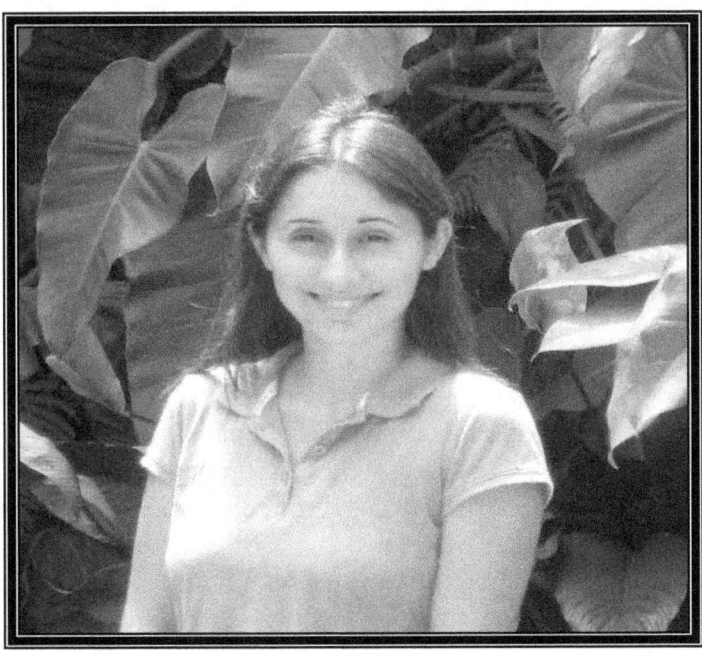

Creating Your Birth

Many people are becoming aware of the basic natural laws of creation in the Universe. My goal is to assist women in using these laws to create more desirable birth experiences. Part of creating the experience you desire will be educating yourself about all of your options. Your options are what you say they are. If you wish to experience home birth you will find a way. If you wish to have a birth center or hospital birth you will also find a way. Think about who will be there with you. What might you be wearing? What will you be saying and hearing? What are the sensations you will experience? Will you want silence upon the baby emerging? Will you keep the cord intact until delivery of the placenta? What other things do you want for you and your baby?

I want you to take some time and think about what you expect to happen. What do you imagine afterward you would say? The reason for this is when I was collecting stories for my book: *Embracing Birth: A Collection of Inspiring Birth Stories* I was able to see the amazing power of belief in action. Many times a mother would say "I knew this would happen" "I told people that this would happen". They may or may not be aware but those things they "knew" would happen did happen because they expected and believed that they would. This is great if it was something they desired, but not so great for things that were bad. Consider thinking things like: I knew I would have a great birth because of all of the love I poured into my baby.

I recommend that you use the 3x a day approach for maximum effectiveness. Morning, noon and night take a moment to create your birth. Your subconscious mind will be overloaded with these amazing new images and thoughts about what you wish to experience. Imagine your birth exactly how you would love for it to be. Write out your birth story how you want to experience it and read it once a day. Write out all of your fears and burn them. Have beautiful affirmations written on flash cards to look at regularly and when labor comes to remind you. Imagine the faces of the people in your company during labor. Hear the loving supportive words they are speaking to you. Learn self hypnosis through hypno-babies or other hypnosis programs. Read positive loving birth stories of other women who have created desirable outcomes. Watch videos of beautiful births to help your visualization processes. Create a vision board of your dream birth and baby. Imagine it in your mind over and over. Feel good, smile, laugh and bring joy to the images. Affirm your belief in your baby and your body's ability to work together in harmony. Imagine the perfect outcome. Have complete faith that this process is bringing you to the perfect end result you desire.

When we take responsibility for our thoughts and for our lives amazing things begin to happen. We are able to experience miracles by having faith in ourselves. You are the ultimate co-creator of your universe and your experience. You can create the labor and birth of your dreams. Birth can be amazing, it can be pain-free and it can be exactly what you want it to be.

Jessica L. Levesque

Please visit my website for loads of resources and information
www.EmbracingBirthBook.com

Afterward

Please seek the advice and care of your health care provider. I am not a Doctor or medical professional.

I hope you enjoyed Embracing Birth: A Collection of Inspiring Birth Stories. Please feel free to contact me with any questions or comments. The following is some general information that I found while doing my own research. I believe each and every parent should do his or her own research into what is best for their family. It's actually better to do your own research because you will learn so much more. Most of the information is geared towards hospital births. This if for a few reasons: If you are having a hospital birth you need to be much more informed as a consumer. Also in only the United States only 25 states have legal midwifery licensing.

Many birth professionals agree it is best to wait as long as you can before you go to the hospital. If you get there too early in your labor it is more likely the hospital will intervene with your labor to "speed things up" and pitocin usually makes things very painful for you and the baby. If you get an epidural to deal with this induced pain the baby will still feel these intense contractions. Epidurals carry many risks so do your research. It is very helpful to let your body do what it needs to do in its own time as long as mom and baby are both doing well. If you want to you can eat once you start labor and drink whatever you want while you are home. You will need lots of energy and staying hydrated is very important. Most hospitals restrict what you can have to clear fluids only even in a long labor. Hire a birth doula or look for a volunteer birth doula. A doula is a childbirth assistant who is invaluable to a laboring woman. She mothers the mother and is educated about various techniques and labor support.

The vitamin K shot is not usually necessary it makes a hole in your baby that he could get an infection from (Hospitals have more germs than any other place). It has not been proven to work. Also breast-fed babies develop vitamin K within eight days of birth on their own. Unless the baby is injured in an accident he does not need it and in that case they would give him the shot. The ointment for the baby's eyes is needed if you have the STD gonorrhea. You can write it in your birth plan that the baby is not to have any of this if it is your wish. Sometimes they may try to give baby a pacifier or sugar water in the nursery, which can interfere with breastfeeding. Putting a sign on the baby's bassinet saying not to do this is can be very helpful.

Please be cautious if you feel you are developing Post-partum depression or during pregnancy depression/anxiety please seek help from a qualified support person. I know personally how difficult this can be. Living a healthy lifestyle with good nutrition can help reduce your risk. Always make time for yourself and you will be a better parent for it.

Vaginal birth after cesarean is your right. Please seek out more information to educate and empower you. ICAN chapters around the USA http://www.ican-online.org Many women are believe that just because they have had a prior c-section they are required to have a repeat. That is not true. I believe in women and their ability to give birth vaginally.

If your baby is breech you can see an acupuncturist for moxi-bustion. You can also see a chiropractor for the Webster technique. Both techniques are very effective in turning breech babies. Babies can also be born breech vaginally safely with an experienced birth professional. If you have to go to the Farm in Tn. Circumcision: Keeping our baby boys intact. Please keep your baby boy intact there is NO medical reason to cut them. Loads of resources on my site about this.

Delayed cord-clamping means not cutting the cord until it is done pulsating. By delaying cord-clamping until the placenta is delivered you ensure the baby gets all of the nutrients and there brain isn't deprived of oxygen. This should always be done long as it is safe for mother and baby. This ensures the baby gets all of the nutrients and has a chance to switch over to breathing oxygen properly. If you do not wish to vaccinate your child and you live in American in the majority of states you can get waivers from the health dept. So if you wish your children can go to daycare and school unvaccinated.

You can look for moms on social networking sites like MySpace, face book, cafe mom and other sites. There may be weekly breastfeeding meet-ups around you check with your local LLL. Story time at the library is a great to meet other parents. You may want to form a group of your own online or join a local moms group. If there are no local groups you can start your own forum for free at www.ning.com and recruit moms at local parks when you are playing with your child.

Breastfeeding information and support. Breast is best for a full year or longer: it is all most babies need. Consider nursing longer it has endless benefits for you and baby. You may like to look into the benefits of child-led weaning as well. If your baby has Jaundice he may need just breast milk and sunlight. Check with your child's doctor. If your supply gets low it can be helpful to stay relaxed as possible and not supplement. If you supplement you may create a stressful cycle because the baby is not requesting your body create more milk. Mother's milk tea helps to and pumping as often as possible will help increase your supply. Make sure to drink plenty of water. Nursing bras are usually a good price on eBay. Your breasts may be very big for the first few months so buying cheap bras is a good idea because once your supply evens out your breasts won't be so large and you will be losing weight because breastfeeding usually makes you lose weight quicker! Baby wearing is great to keep baby close and comfy while moving about. Breastfeeding is not birth control! Study after study shows the benefits of breast milk for both the mom and baby yet only 12% of American mothers exclusively breastfeed until 6 months.

You can take the mini pill after six weeks post partum. If you do not wait the six weeks to have sex please keep lots of lube on hand or you may regret it. There are also spermicidal films which offer a great non hormonal alternative that you can buy at most pharmacies.

You can buy Poise panties in the Depends section. They are perfect for the first few weeks after birth you won't have to worry about messes on your sheets. You may only need one pack they are about $12 at Wal-Mart and are very comfy. It is very helpful to use the peri bottle to wash every time you go to the bathroom. Sits baths are when you soak your bottom in witch hazel and warm/hot water for 15 minutes as many times a day as possible to relieve any discomfort. If you get hemorrhoids you can buy cotton pads for a dollar and witch hazel and soak them put them in a wet wipes tub. If you are having discomfort you can wet some wash cloths and put them in little snack sandwich baggies and freeze them they will feel really nice when applied to the perineum.

Restorative mothers multivitamins are available. When you are ready to begin exercising do something fun that you love to do 3x a week. Eat a healthy well balanced diet and go out there and have fun. Life can be fun! Always follow your heart in parenting and look within for the answers within. Take it easy and enjoy your baby moon. Restore your body mind and soul. Accept help and feel the love.   Rejoice in your amazing body. Give to yourself love until you overflow. Tell everyone how amazing birth can be and help other moms any way you can. We are all in this together. Have a great birth!

Best wishes,
Jessica Levesque

www.EmbracingBirthBook.com
www.Myspace.com/EmbracingBirth
www.Youtube.com/BirthingWise
 Jessica@EmbracingBirthBook.com

Birth Resources

Finding a Doula or Midwife:
http://www.birthpartners.com
www.doula.com
www.ACNM.org
www.cfmidwifery.org
http://www.childbirthprofessional.com
http://www.birthingfromwithin.com
www.DONA.org
www.doulaworld.com
http://www.socalbirth.org
http://www.flmidwifery.org

ADVOCACY & BIRTH RESOURCES
Childbirth Connection: 212.777.5000 - www.childbirthconnection.org
Choices In Childbirth: 212.983.4122 - www.choicesinchildbirth.org
Citizens for Midwifery: 888.CFM.4880 - www.cfmidwifery.org
My Birth Team - www.mybirthteam.com
Birth Works: 888.TO.BIRTH - www.birthworks.org
Coalition for Improving Maternity Services (CIMS) - www.motherfriendly.org
American Association of Birth Centers (AABC) - www.birthcenters.org
Perinatal Education Associates - www.birthsource.com
Birth Policy: The Big Push for Midwives - www.birthpolicy.org

CHILDBIRTH EDUCATION
Birthing from Within: 505.254.4884 - www.birthingfromwithin.com
The Bradley Method: 800.4.A.BIRTH - www.bradleybirth.com
Lamaze International: 800.368.4404 - www.lamaze.org
HypnoBirthing: 603.798.3286 - www.hypnobirthing.com
HypnoBabies: 714.952.2229 - www.hypnobabies.com

MIDWIVES PROFESSIONAL ORGANIZATIONS
American College of Nurse-Midwives: 240.485.1800 - www.acnm.org
Midwives Alliance of North America (MANA): 888.923.MANA (6262) - www.mana.org
American Midwifery Certification Board (AMCB) - www.amcbmidwife.org
DOULAS
Assoc. of Labor Assistants & Childbirth Educators (ALACE): 888.222.5223 - www.alace.org
Doulas of North America (DONA) International: 888.788.DONA (3662) - www.dona.org
CESAREANS
International Cesarean Awareness Network, Inc. (ICAN) - www.ican-online.org
The Business of Being Born: http://thebusinessofbeingborn.com/
Birth as We Know It: http://www.birthasweknowit.com/
Birth in America: http://www.youtube.com/watch?v=R3WWNKurKjA

Embracing Birth: A Collection of Inspiring Birth Stories

Recommended reading
A Thinking Woman's Guide to a Better Birth by Henci Goer
Ian May's Guide to Childbirth by Ian May Gaskin
Spiritual Midwifery by Ian May Gaskin
Very Brave and Courageous: The Vaginal Birth after Cesarean Experience by Lynn Baptisti Richards.
Sit up and Take Notice by Pauline Scott
Homebirth: The Essential Guide to Giving Birth Outside of The Hospital by Sheila Kitzinger
Special Delivery: The Complete Guide to Informed Birth by Rahima Baldwin
Open Season by Nancy Cohen is specific to VBAC and natural childbirth.
Cesarean Section: Understanding and Celebrating Your Baby's Birth by Michele C. Moore and Caroline M. De Costa
Active Birth by Janet Balaskas
Natural Childbirth the Bradley Way by Erick Ingraham, and Robert A. Bradley
The Birth Partner by Penny Simkin
Birth Without Violence by Frederick Leboyer
Gentle Birth Choices by Barbara Harper and Suzanne Arms
A Good Birth, A Safe Birth Choosing and Having the Childbirth Experience You Want by Diana Korte
Immaculate Deception II Myth Magic and Birth by Suzanne Arms
Birth Reborn by Michael Odent
What If I Have a C-Section? By Rita Rubin
Reclaiming the Spirituality of Birth by Benig Mauger
The Caesarean by Michael Odent
HypnoBirthing the Mongan Method by Marie F. Mongan
This is a great way to relax for the VBAC uterus.
Artemis Speaks: V.B.A.C. Stories & Natural Childbirth Information by Nan Koehler
Born in the USA: How a Broken Maternity System Must Be Fixed to Put Women and Children First by Marsden Wagner
Jennifer Gianni's Fusion Pilates for Post Pregnancy & C-Section Recovery by Jennifer Gianni
Natural Childbirth After Cesarean: A practical Guide by Karis Crawford & Johanne C. Walters
PUSHED: The Painful Truth About Childbirth And Modern Maternity Care by Jennifer Block. There is a chapter titled "Denied Birth" that covers the issues of vaginal breech birth and VBAC very well.
Birthing From Within by Pam England

Thank you to all the birth professionals who are dedicated to supporting and educating mothers and fathers. Together we can change the world one birth at a time.

Jessica Levesque

www.ingramcontent.com/pod-product-compliance
Lightning Source LLC
Chambersburg PA
CBHW051956280526
45793CB00005B/738